THE FUNDAMENTAL THEORY OF DIABETES DISORDER

About the author:

Mr GODWIN MILLINGTON.

Diabetes Specialist in LTC Clinical Dpt.

Phlebotomist in Primary Healthcare.

BSC Hons Nursing and Midwifery 2010.

BSC Hons In Diabetes Genomic, Aetiology and Intervention.

THE FUNDAMENTAL THEORY OF DIABETES DISORDER

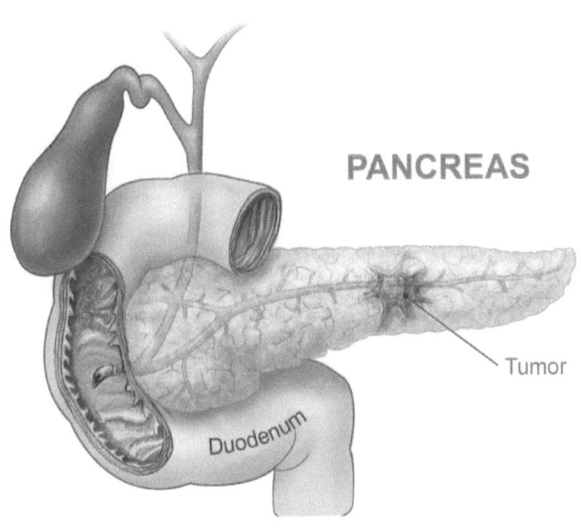

GODWIN MILLINGTON

Published by New Generation Publishing in 2020

Copyright © Godwin Millington 2020

First Edition

The author asserts the moral right under the Copyright, Designs and Patents Act 1988 to be identified as the author of this work.

All Rights reserved. No part of this publication may be reproduced, stored in a retrieval system or transmitted, in any form or by any means without the prior consent of the author, nor be otherwise circulated in any form of binding or cover other than that in which it is published and without a similar condition being imposed on the subsequent purchaser.

ISBN: 978-1-80031-986-8

www.newgeneration-publishing.com
New Generation Publishing

Contents

Introduction 1
   The Epidemiology of Diabetes and Statistics 2
   What Is Pancreas and Diabetes 6
What is Pre-diabetes 10
What is Diabetes 17
   What is Type 1 Diabetes 23
   What is type 2 diabetes 28
   The difference between type 1 and type 2 diabetes 33
   What causes diabetes type 1 and type 2 33
   Gestational diabetes 38
Diabetes Management 46
   Risk Factors leading to diabetes. 60
Complications Of Diabetes 67
   Microvascular Complication of Diabetes, Eye, Kidney, nerve disease 67
   Macrovascular complications of diabetes, Heart, brain and blood vessels 72
Prevention of Diabetes 72
What Is The Treatment For Diabetes 84
What is Hyperglycaemia 93
Hypoglycaemia of Diabetes 96
Summary 101

INTRODUCTION

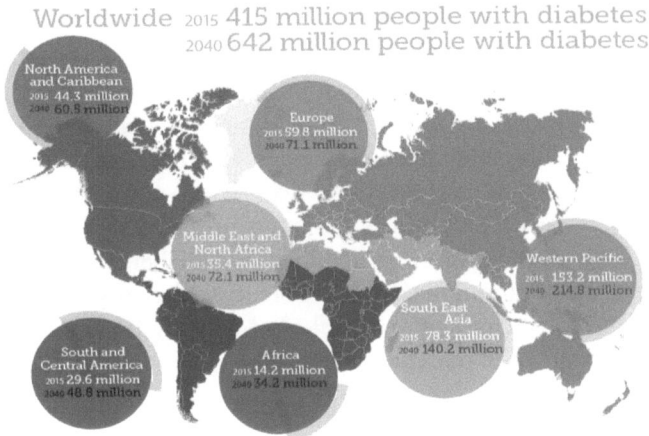

Guideline Of Diabetes Worldwide

Diabetes is a common disease that affects 425 million people both in America, UK and worldwide and there are 197 million under diagnosis that do not even know they have the disorder, according to the WHO Organisation and according to new report who said that as from last year's estimate, 516 million people had the disease. While 5 million people died from diabetes in 2014, by 2040 the research estimated 650 million people will suffer from the disease and while others millions of undiagnosed people who develop diabetes complications are noted. The world is expected to see morbidity and mortality to be reduced from diabetes disorder, because of early diagnosis. Why do will called diabetes mellitus and where the word diabetes comes from. In Greek language and this means a "siphon" Aretus the Cappadocia, according to Greek physician during the second century A.D the name and condition was given diabainein. He used the word to described patients who were passing too much water or urine like a siphon. The word became "diabetes" from the English language adoption of the Medieval Latin diabetes. In 1674, Thomas Willis added mellitus to the term called diabetes mellitus, although it is commonly referred to simply as diabetes. Mel in Latin means "honey"; the urine and blood of people with diabetes has excess glucose, and the word glucose means is sweet like honey. Diabetes mellitus could accurately mean The 'siphoning off sweet'. According to recent research who also said that diabetes cannot be cure, but can be manageable and is advised that with good control, management of diabetes is essential to avoid developing long and short term complications and diabetes can also reverse back automatically by itself if you're in good diet plan, but some can't be reversible, but with medication your diabetes can be under control.

The Epidemiology of Diabetes and Statistics

The incidence of diabetes all three types of diabetes is estimated roughly 5% in the worldwide and it's also predicted that there may be a further 3% of the people with undiagnosed or unknown diabetes still roaming round and a recent research also commented about related incidence of diabetic patients in the UK and worldwide by classification of type 1 DM 35% of cases type 2 DM 70% of cases types 3 DM 5% of cases are finding.

Morbidity of Diabetes

Diabetes cause lots of complications to the sufferers in our society today and people who are been diagnosis with diabetes in any age group 40-64 years are 20 times more likely to be recorded blind than the non-diabetic patients of the same age. Diabetic retinopathy is one of the lead causes of blindness in worldwide today and diabetes also affects other part of the body according to recent research who said that up to 40% of people who are early diagnosis of type 1 diabetes before the age of 30 years are undergoing a diabetes related nephropathy, renal failure, neuropathy, which can cause lot of complication issues including from foot ulceration, sexual difficulties, cardiac and sudden death.

Mortality of Diabetes

According to world health organisation (WHO) who stated that 30,000 people per year die prematurely because of diabetes disorder and the cost of these deaths are mostly from the macrovascular and microvascular complications such as myocardial infarcts and cerebrovascular accidents, stroke, nephropathy. The new research also emphasises that a number of people found death prematurely is know as diabetic complication is double of non-diabetic population worldwide.

The Aetiology of Diabetes

The Aetiology of type 1 and type 2 means the fundamental causes or the origin of the disease and the major factors which base on family predisposition toward the life illness and meanwhile type 1 diabetes is always present in the teens with a short history of weight loss, thirst, passing lots of urine and such patients or child are often thin and in some cases there is no family or genetic history of diabetes. Although the cause of the chronic illness is unknown or could be the pancreas is defected and failure could be triggered by a viral infection and autoimmune disorder during childhood. Type 2 diabetes is also present later in life from 40 to 50 years of age and some time it suddenly happen when your lifestyles change or body mass index overweight and other cases there is often a strong family history that contributed to type 2 diabetes disorder.

Coping with the Diagnosis

Is a shock to both child and parents who are been diagnosis with chronic diabetes disorder and family has a different reactions after diagnosis with diabetes and in a short time most children and families go through a grieving time with the onset of the illness. Both feel bad about the broken sad news from the test result and some time from the shock they also feel denial, sad, anxiety, fear, anger, and guilt, while suddenly they have diagnosis with diabetes disorder in the family and with short time families do adjust and get on with life or adapted to diabetes and self-control management plan.

Can Diabetes Be Cure

According to world health organisation (WHO) in 2018 and some others researcher who also stated that no cure for diabetes, but sometime it can be automatically reversible by itself or depend how complication issues is base. The circle of lifestyle and genetic predisposition of diabetes, there is no guarantee that it would automatically reverse back due to the response of the growing health burden of diabetes mellitus today and the UK diabetes and the community have figure three choices how to secure diabetes in good other, include prevention of diabetes, managing diabetes, and take better care of the people with diabetes to allowed them to prevent the onset of diabetes complications. All three mentions are helpful to prevent the risk and management of diabetes and the recommended approaches are actively being pursued by the Department of Health, Human Services today and public health.

How prevalent is diabetes among population

According to WHO that majority of black people are 1.9 times likely to develop diabetes than white population, but the prevalence of diabetes among black people has quadrupled during the past thirty-four years ago and meanwhile among black people age twenty and older is about 3.5 million have diabetes worldwide. The WHO also stated that the global prevalence of diabetes among adults over 18 years of age has risen from 5.9% in 2015 to 9.5% in 2018 and meanwhile diabetes prevalence has been declared rising more rapidly day to day in middle class and lower income countries also contributed to the rise of the onset of diabetes in the world. The world knows that diabetes complication is a major cause of blindness, kidney failure, heart attacks, stroke and lower limb amputation which lead to premature death over the years and while the death rates of the people black with diabetes are 35 percent higher than white's majority or population in worldwide.

Emotional Effects of Diabetes

Diabetes can take it's toll on you every blessed day, your psychological, emotional wellbeing and other negative though can take it place on high blood glucose monitor and diabetes itself affected your body more than blood sugar and it can suddenly lead to mood changes in personal relationships. The physiology and psychology effect of diabetes may lead you anxiety, nervous and confusion in your personal life, because stress of living with diabetes which can contribute to changes of your mood due to high glucose level. Mood and emotional struggle is quite difficult for family, friend to understand your mood swings and you also need a support group to help you promote stronger healthier relationship and to reduce the risk that attached to diabetes disorder.

The Circle of Diabetes

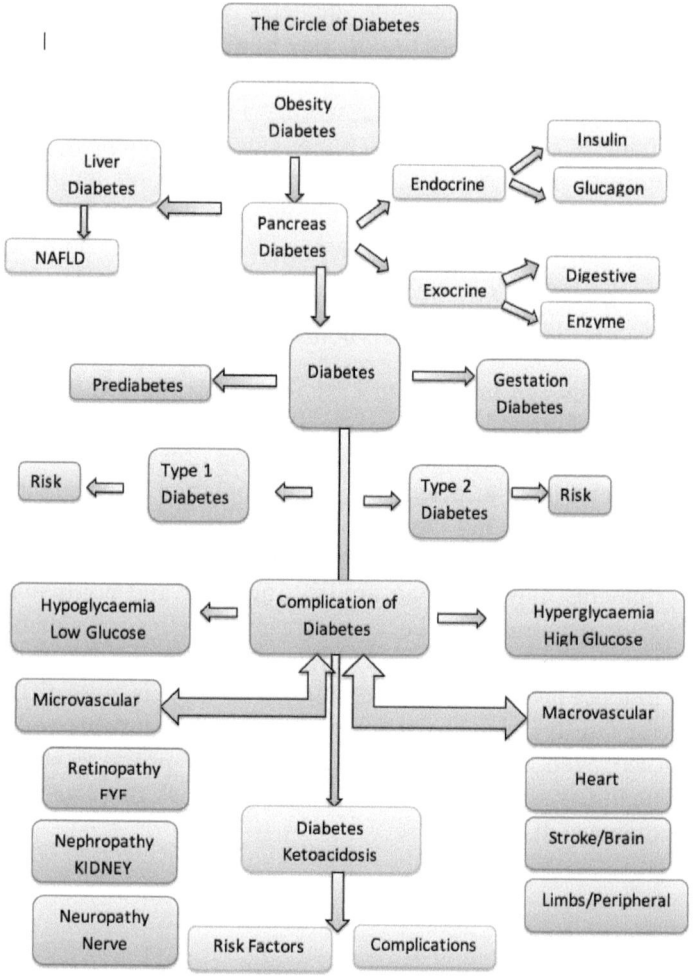

What Is Pancreas and Diabetes

Pancreas is a long soft organ located in abdomen behind the lower part of your posterior abdominal wall and stomach which plays an important role in diabetes disorder. Pancreas is the organ that produces insulin, calls hormones that helps to digest food in the body because all parts of your body need glucose for energy used and glucose refers to sugar levels in your body system and while each cell in your body needs glucose as energy use.

When pancreas disorder is damage it can't or doesn't make use of it functions any more, them the glucose will build up in the bloodstream and leave the cells to be starved for energy demand and if too much blood glucose build up in your bloodstream it cause complication calls hyperglycaemia and the symptoms include thirsty, nausea and shortness of breath. When someone has a low blood glucose level which known as hypoglycaemia can cause many symptoms, including shakiness, dizziness and loss of consciousness and hypoglycaemia can be a life threatening to someone with diabetes disorder. However neglected to control diabetes disorder will be at risk of complication.

Pancreas also plays two different roles in the management of the body insulin systems, which are **Endocrine and Exocrine system.**

The endocrine system

The endocrine system is the organs that produce chemicals hormones that regulate and transported metabolism through the bloodstream to help regulate growth of our body and endocrine also responsible for the growing, mood, sexual function and reproduction process and there are also others two type of hormones produced by the pancreas which are **insulin and glucagon.** While insulin acts to lower your blood sugar level and glucagon which also acts to high or balance your blood sugar level to maintained all the function of your organs including brain, kidneys and liver.

The exocrine system

Exocrine system is an organ that produces a number of glands that release substances in the body such as saliva, sweat and glands within the gastrointestinal track and in this process there are digestive enzymes involved in releasing substance, lipase to break down fats. These happened when food enters the stomach, the pancreatic fluids or juice supply by bile are released into the ducts through duodenum (intestine) and the **gallbladder** produces digestive fluid called **bile** that is released into the duodenum which help the body to digest carbohydrate, proteins and fats into the body, but with the people suffering of type 1 or 2 diabetes there is no other possibility to make used of this substance that is supplied by gallbladder.

What role does the pancreas play in diabetes

Type 1 diabetes
With type 1 diabetes the immune system terminates the pancreas's beta cells that supply insulin or energy to the body and that is the reason while type 1 can no longer produce insulin to the bloodstream as energy use and with setting time the body becomes starved for lack of energy, because the body needs insulin to survive the journey and during these process the body start demanded and the body becomes insulin resistant.

Type 2 diabetes
With type 2 diabetes, the pancreas manage to produces little insulin to the body, but not enough to serve or run as body energy, meanwhile the body doesn't equally respond to the little insulin that is supplied as it should be and while the muscle, fat and liver cell never respond to insulin correctly, because there is insulin resistance, the beta cells of the pancreas's islets can no longer keep

up with the body's demand for insulin to lower blood glucose to normal levels which is called (glucagon).

In this process the pancreas is strongly to produce enough insulin to enable control down sugar levels, while then the symptoms of diabetes become visible or appearing to see the clinic for more investigation.

The cause of pancreas disorder

- Excessive alcohol use
- Gallstones
- High triglyceride levels in the blood
- High calcium levels in the blood
- Lack of Physical inactivity
- Poor diet
- Ageing
- Obesity
- Genetic

What is Prediabetes

Prediabetes is a process whereby the amount of glucose (sugar) in the bloodstream is higher than normal range, but not high enough to be diagnosing as diabetes type 2, but at this junction you are at risks of develop types 2 diabetes. With more effort and help of physical activity, exercise and weight loss plan, life style change would help preventing the onset of type 2 diabetes disorder in the nearest future. Prediabetes is also a warning sign that without taking the nest steps to change your risks of develop type 2 diabetes would result in a serious problem of chronic disorder. Most people with prediabetes experience warning sign that can lead to type 2 diabetes, sometime can be self-negligent toward the onset of diabetes and meanwhile prediabetes are a gradually high risk of progressive to type 2 with heart condition and other health issues. Prediabetes can be prevented by reducing your lifestyle change and return to healthier eating habits or diets. Daily physical activities which can be a huge benefit to your blood glucose balance levels without doctor intervention or medication recommendation.

How did I get prediabetes

There are three main things that can cause prediabetes in your life without progression into type 2 diabetes and in other hand there is something you can't change regardless to your genetics predispose, but you can help yourself to lower your eating habits against fat foods and calories consumption to improve your daily physical activity. It is vital to realised that when person is prediabetes disorder this not a question of not eating sugar or eating less sugar, but is your body's pancreas ability to produce insulin at that moment to other part of the body cell to use as energy. With thyroid problem this can also linked to prediabetes issues, because thyroid infection it's hard to keep or regulate normal weight balance and being overweight would affects the body's mass ability to circulate blood sugar level round into the bloodstream. Advice, Watch what you do and eat and long periods of stay home setting in one place laziness, would reduce the circulation of insulin (sugar) to all part of the body as energy use.

How do we prevent prediabetes

If prediabetes problem can be detect earlier on and it can be reversed back or can be prevented into full type 2 diabetes disorder, because in worldwide, 7 % to 10% of people who was previously diagnosed with prediabetes lead to type 2 diabetes without follow up the recommendation advice from doctor. There are others principle factors for consideration including, changes of your diet and daily physical exercise and also to change your lifestyle would be a great better for your blood glucose level to return to normal range.

The causes of prediabetes

The main cause of prediabetes is unknown and what we do known according to many researchers who emphasis on family history, lifestyles, age, overweight, lack of exercise and genetics predisposed which play an important part of your predicament of prediabetes is lack of physical activity and excessive fat abdominal, also seem to be significant factors which contributed to prediabetes disorder. Prediabetes can be progressive when your body start to develop problem using the hormone called insulin, because insulin is the only one transporting your glucose round to your body to use as energy through your bloodstream. If you have been diagnosed with prediabetes this means your body can't produce enough insulin at this time, this is what we called insulin resistance and insulin resistance means your bodies build up too much glucose in your blood cell which can lead to high normal glucose reading on your body.

Symptoms of prediabetes

Prediabetes develops gradually when your blood glucose is higher than normal range by not experience sign and symptoms at all and prediabetes is called silent killer condition, because it has no sign and symptoms. The prediabetes stay in your body for several years without knowing it and is only common risk factor can exposed or trigger out the symptomatic or several test to carried the cause of the problem. At this moment or situation is better for you to see your doctor if you're concerned about family history of diabetes, obese or if you experience a warning sign related symptoms.

Symptoms

- Hungry than normal
- Weight losing
- Thirsty
- Frequent urine
- Fatigue
- Blurred vision
- Family history
- High cholesterol
- Being 35/40 year older

Diagnoses

Diagnosis is taken place when doctor seen you are overweight, losing weight, eyes vision blurred, the blood test is requested by GP for fasting glucose test or HbA1c and body mass index BMI when is over 27, this happened when you have one or more risk factors that can cause the onset of prediabetes. The doctor can also use the same blood test to carry out type 2 diabetes tests to know if you are positive for cholesterol/ triglycerides glucose level test after 8 hours of not eating which is preferable to be done in the morning after overnight fasting sleep. When blood routine result levels raise higher or lower than as usual is called abnormal result test and this can carry out in the following process called.

Fasting plasma glucose test (FPG) fast this is a method used to screening for diabetes and is also use to measure blood glucose level for people with symptoms of diabetes and test to be carried out with overnight fasting after blood test if the result of the glucose level is still in high position or more than 7.0mmoll/l then you will consider to be develop prediabetes and sometime you may hear doctor used a phrase word impaired fasting glucose.

Fasting Glucose test
Normal – 4.0 / 6.0mmol/L
Prediabetes –6-0 / 8.0mmol/L or higher

Oral glucose tolerance test (OGTT) this is another test carried out as prediabetes disorder and this will be fasting blood glucose level and you will asked to drink 75g of sugary mixture and two hours later your blood glucose will be measure. After the test, if your blood glucose is more than 200mg/DL with tolerance test you may presume you have developed diabetes disorder.

Oral glucose tolerance test
Normal – Below 5.0 TO 6.0 mmol/L
Prediabetes – Between 6.0 TO 7.0 mmol/L
Diabetes – 7.10 TO 8.00 mmol/L or higher

The Treatment for Prediabetes

The treatment for prediabetes is used to help prevent the onset of a full type 2 diabetes and the effective of the treatment for prediabetes is a weight loose, lifestyle change and regular exercise can help to improve insulin resistant and lower your blood glucose level. In many cases exercise and daily activity help circulate your insulin round your body system and to prevent develop type 2 diabetes and in the beginning drug called metformin is used to help lower your blood glucose levels first and lower the risk of develop diabetes complication and some others common treatment is as follow.

Eating well. A dietician or certified diabetes educator can also help you for your meal plan that is good for your blood glucose level and the purpose of a meal plan is to have a control of your blood glucose level and keep yourself healthier.

Exercise. The more you do exercise the more your glucose is in balance circulation glucose around your body to becomes less resistant to insulin and little of exercise also improve your blood glucose level, According to British and America diabetes association who recommended that every 30 minute of moderate physical activity a day it's would help to prevent the onset of diabetes.

Lose weight. Being overweight is one of the primary risk factor for prediabetes and the more fatty tissue in your body, the more the risk you develop diabetes, especially in between the muscle and skin around your abdomen which lead to more resistant to insulin. Soon as you have your diagnosis result as positive and at that moment someone start to prepared yourself to lose weight or start loss weight program immediately, because losing weight of 6-10% can help contribute a significant risk reduction of developing type 2 diabetes disorder.

Metformin. Metformin should be used for people who has type 2 diabetes after result or being diagnosed with diabetes the doctor may recommended a medication that will prevent the onset of diabetes complication to reduce your glucose level. Medication prescription metformin is used to prevent type 2 diabetes to keep the liver from producing more glucose when you don't need it and keep your blood glucose level in orders.

Waist size. A large waist size can provoke insulin resistance to lower your glucose flowing through your body stream and it will increase the risk of insulin resistance to goes up for men with waists larger than 42 inches and for women with waists larger than 38 inches.

Dietary patterns. By eating red meat or beef or drinking sugary sweetened stuff can associate with a higher risk of prediabetes development and a diet high in fruits, nuts, vegetables, olive oil and whole grains associated in reducing your risk of develop a complication of diabetes or can also help to prevent lower risk of prediabetes disorder.

Inactivity.
The less daily activity you do, the greater your risk of develop prediabetes are in order and while physical activity helps you control your weight, uses up glucose as energy and makes your cells more sensitive to insulin.

Age. According to WHO said that diabetes can develop at any age, the risk of prediabetes increases after 35 to 50 year of age and due to lack of regular exercise, life change or eating more than 3000 calories a day can put you at risk.

How serious is prediabetes

Prediabetes is a thoughtful matter to your health and this means that you are at middle risk of develop type 2 diabetes and diabetes risk if not withdrawing from your lifestyle, meanwhile some action need to be taken just to avoid complication of diabetes. In many cases 35-100 who are prediabetes will progressing to type 2 diabetes within the next three years and other hand if your local GP test result has been consider the levels of glucose tolerance if higher than normal can being predicted to have diabetes in the future. Heart risk, for whoever develop prediabetes or type 2 diabetes often have high blood pressure in the future and also twice as likely to develop cardiovascular disease, heart attack, angina and stroke from diabetes complication. The result also based on a number of risk factors of a smoker, cholesterol, ages and blood pressure should be follow to prevent the risk of develop premature heart attack or death.

What Is Diabetes?

Diabetes is a chronic metabolic disease and is a lifelong disease that occurs when the pancreas does not produce enough insulin or when the body cannot convert glucose as energy use and diabetes is known as a condition that is affected the body when the body can't longer used the insulin it produces as energy. What insulin does, insulin is a hormone that regulates blood sugar level in your body and insulin helps transport blood glucose to all part of your body's cells and lowers the amount of sugar level in your bloodstream. Meanwhile, If a person is diabetic that mean your body doesn't make enough insulin or insulin it produce doesn't work properly, the bodies rejected your insulin and the insulin glucose that formulate in your bloodstream become high and chances to reach your cells to serve as energy use is block. Glucose (sugar) is absorbed into the bloodstream, where it enters cells with the help of insulin and while liver stores and produces a standard glucose to the bloodstream. Meanwhile if a blood glucose levels are very low, because you haven't been eaten for short time, the liver breaks down stored glycogen into glucose to keep your glucose level within a normal range and with diabetes patients the insulin would not supplied enough glucose to the body to use as energy, them it become insulin resistance. A chronic diabetes is considered as a group of defected disease how your body use blood glucose on your system, because sugar level is essential to your health wise and is also known as a source of energy to your cell muscles and tissues and also provide your brain as a fuel supplied. The cause of different type of diabetes is varied and depend the type of diabetes you have been diagnoses with and each can lead to high glucose in your bloodstream, because too much sugar in your body can provoke a serious health problems. The defected diabetes condition include prediabetes, type 1 and type 2 and some other group are potentially reversible condition such as prediabetes is when your blood glucose are higher than normal reading, but it consider not high sufficient to pronounce as full diabetes and gestational diabetes which known as pregnancy disorder, but can be reversible after birth.

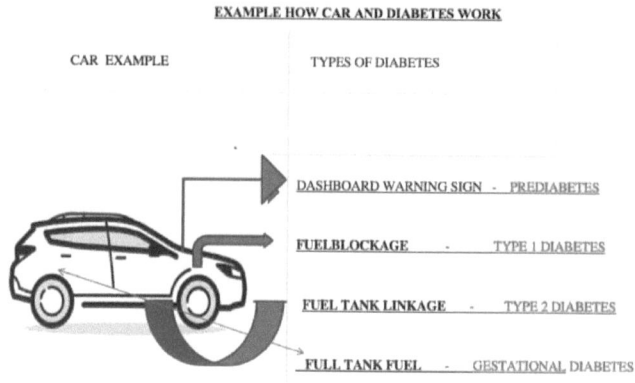

EXAMPLE HOW CAR AND DIABETES WORK

CAR EXAMPLE — TYPES OF DIABETES

DASHBOARD WARNING SIGN - PREDIABETES

FUELBLOCKAGE - TYPE 1 DIABETES

FUEL TANK LINKAGE - TYPE 2 DIABETES

FULL TANK FUEL - GESTATIONAL DIABETES

What Is The Prognosis Of Diabetes?

The prognosis of diabetes is connected to the degree in which the situation is under control to prevent the onset of diabetes for a long-term complications and some of the long-term complications is to prevented, kidney failure and cardiovascular disease or stroke which can be life threatening. The acute complications such as diabetic ketoacidosis can be life threatening to someone with diabetes and with help of your blood sugar levels control may delayed the onset of complications, and in the UK or worldwide so many people who has been diagnosis with diabetes disorder leave their lives successful. The prognosis of diabetes can also reduce life expectancy and these diseases can also be monitored or controlled by you with the help of your lifestyle change.

The prognosis of prediabetes is about 10% spread or chance of develop into type 2 diabetes which can occur within years without knowing it and the chances of developing type 2 diabetes in life time is greater to 80% in the average population. But improving yourself with dietary food and regular exercise can help prevent the onset of type 2 diabetes in the nearest future, according to the new researcher who said that weight loss of 6% and regular 30 minute exercise daily reduce the risk of diabetes disorder by 50% upward.

Target blood glucose set by healthcare team is to fall below

TARGET BY TYPE	LEVEL	BEFORE MEAL	AT LEAST 120 MINUTE AFTER MEAL
Non-Diabetic		4.0 to 7.0 mmol/l	Under 6.0 to 8.0mmol
Type 2 diabetes		4.0 to 7.0mmol/l	8.0 to 15.0mmol/l
Type 1 Diabetes	5 to 8mmol/l	4.0 to 7.0mmol/l	10.0 t0 15.0mmol
Children with type 1 diabetes	4 to 8 mmol/l	4.0 to 7.0mmol/l	6.0 to 10.0mmol/l

Diagnosed of Diabetes

The diagnosis of diabetes can be carried out in a simple blood test measuring depend on the level of your blood glucose reading and symptoms because the diagnose of diabetes does not wait for inconvenient time in life and usually these tests result are repeatable on a subsequent day to confirm the final diagnosis before doctor would decide to put you on medication or self-diet program. A diagnosis of diabetes is also a frightening and threating to life spam and family expectation can place a huge enormous emotional, financial burden on this illness and yourself or people mine feel anxious of their result, because it may come as a shock to that person or personal matter. People with type 1 and type 2 diabetes may hear their condition described as "mild, but any diabetes disorder is not a "mild" medical report and all diabetes person are serious condition and life threating, because it goes with sort of many complications issues, including (microvascular risk, retinopathy, nerve neuropathy, nerve, eye, and kidney damage and while the risk of (macrovascular) can causes stroke, cardio CVD) this is most complication of heart and stroke diseases.

Why is it important to avoid diabetes

Because diabetes is a serious illness it can be a treat or life sentence with medication or insulin injections, but some time with treatment, the condition usually gets worse over time, but could be better with your lifestyle change. The risk of developing short and long-term complication is greater, like heart disease or stroke, eye and nerve is very common than in the rest of the people without diabetes. According to recent researchers who said that people who has been diagnose with diabetes die premature from heart disease or stroke and they also found of develop serious complication issues such as impaired kidney failure, and nerve system. Diabetes is known as one of the leading cause of amputation in the worldwide, but although it can be prevented and monitor to higher degree standard and with good management or control of your blood pressure and blood sugar level will help prevent the onset of complication in life.

How diabetes can causes health problems

In some people who has been diagnoses with type 1 diabetes, who also on treatment are simply develop high blood sugar levels within or during treatment period and the complication within is Hypoglycaemia and hyperglycaemia. Hypoglycaemia is known as condition caused by a very low level of blood sugar (glucose in your body) and when someone is known as a diabetes patient and other variety of conditions can cause low blood sugar in people without diabetes. Immediate treatment of hypoglycaemia is quite necessary when blood sugar levels are very low to 3.4 millimoles per litre (mmol/L) or below and treatment involves in quick steps to get your blood sugar level back into a normal range either you give a high-sugar foods or drinks or with liquid honey drink.

Diabetes hyperglycaemia is known as a high blood sugar condition that affected the people that is suffering of diabetes and several factors can contribute to hyperglycaemia in people with diabetes disorder, including food and lack of physical activity. It's very vital to recognised the treatment of hyperglycaemia according to medical intervention, because if a person left untreated it can become severe and lead to serious complications that requiring emergency care, such as a diabetic coma or death. Several factors can also contribute to hyperglycaemia with people suffering of diabetes, including not eating well and lack of physical activity or others illness, medications, or skipping medication.

What Is Type 1 Diabetes

Type 1 diabetes is chronic disorder in which the pancreas can't longer produce insulin to the body as energy use and type 1 diabetes is also known as autoimmune disease that causes the insulin producing beta cells in the pancreas to be destroyed, and beta cell is organ that prevent the body to able to produce enough insulin that regulate blood glucose levels. Due to the destruction of beta cells has been damaged and the body is unable to produce any insulin to the cell in the body then the onset of diabetes begin and sometime with type 1 diabetes is known as autoimmune infection whereby the immune system destroys by beta cell in pancreas grand and the onset beginning to appear in childhood or before the adulthood stage. The sign and symptoms happen when the amount of insulin produce to the body is insufficient to use as energy. The insulin in the body is the major key that can unlocks the door to the body's cells and during this process once the door is unlocked glucose can enter the body cells where it is circulate as fuel round the body. In type 1 diabetes the body is unable to produce any insulin, because there is no major key to unlock the door for insulin to circulate round and the glucose start to accumulate or builds up in the bloodstream.

Type 1 diabetes is manifested by the immune system that destroying the beta cells in the pancreas grand that produce insulin to the body and the body immune system attack and destroys own beta cell. What immune system does in the body is to protect the body from dangerous infection or disease is identifying as a destroyed harmful substance during childhood.

Anybody can develop type 1 diabetes in any age, but usually happened early age especially in childhood from 3-6 month or it happened before the age of 15 year with short history of genetic and it often follows a trigger such as a viral infection.

Prognosis of type 1 diabetes

According to researcher who said that the general statistical prognosis of type 1 diabetes is that 18% of sufferers of type 1 diabetes will die before the age of 50 to 65 and in other way there is good researcher who discover that there is less incident or death rate than it, because there are new advances technology and understanding of the disease make things more easier than before and with good monitor of blood sugar control level and a healthy diet can lead to a long life for type 1 sufferers.

Diabetes is equally easy to control with the right medical care, so as acute complications can be avoided which known as long-term complications such as kidney, eye, circulatory system, and nerve fibres are also the most common complication of type 1 diabetes and if left untreated, diabetes can result in complication health issues in coma or early death.

Type 1 symptoms

Type 1 diabetes develops slowly and the symptoms happen suddenly and if anyone has symptoms listed below should be follow up immediately or make an appointment to see the doctor and there are some general absence of public awareness of the sign and symptoms of type 1 diabetes and everyone need to be proactive about your health of any family members who has history of diabetes.

Symptoms

Type 1 diabetes signs and symptoms can appear suddenly and may include:

- Increased thirst
- Frequent urination
- Bed-wetting in children who previously didn't wet the bed during the night
- Extreme hunger
- Unintended weight loss

- Irritability and other mood changes
- Fatigue and weakness
- Blurred vision

The causes and risk factors of type 1 diabetes

Type 1 diabetes is caused by body's immune system by mistakenly targets and kills beta cells in pancreas that responsible for producing insulin to the body as energy, because the more insulin produce into pancreas, the more insulin become resistant to the body and at a time pancreas can no longer control the blood glucose levels, them the symptoms of diabetes begin to appear suddenly. What causes the type 1 diabetes is unknown, however, research suggested that the condition results from a combination of genetic predisposition with an environmental trigger and auto immune system are the main cause. There are many several factors that also contributed to type 1 diabetes and most of the time genetic predisposed can lead to type 1 diabetes immediately and genetic factors is located on chromosome which call HLA human leukocyte antigen complex. One of the causes are as follow.

Viral infections: According to a research who found out that there are certain viruses that can cause the onset of types 1 diabetes by immune system turn against he own body, instead of assisting to fight infection from the body.

Race/ethnicity: A certain ethnicities has contributed to high degree of type 1 diabetes and worldwide are seem to more disposed to type 1 and while some others country like Chinese have a lower risk of develop types 1 and south America.

Geographical location
A certain people who live in northern climate has develop higher risk of develop type 1 diabetes, because

it has been known to certain people live in northern climate, because they are in door during the winter period are less likely to develop type 1.

Family history
Inherited from family or genetic predisposition has proof that link to type 1 diabetes and if you are from gene family there are possibility you will got it or at risk of develop diabetes disorder.

Race
Why people of certain races develop it, including African-Americans, Hispanics, Native Americans, Asian-Americans and Pacific Islanders are more likely to develop prediabetes in their life.

Sleep
People with a certain sleep disorder (obstructive sleep apnoea) have an increased risk of develop prediabetes, because insulin resistance to the body or people who do work changing shifts or night shifts develop prediabetes in respect of short sleep time and other conditions also associated with prediabetes include. High blood pressure. Low levels of high-density lipoprotein (HDL) cholesterol, High levels of triglycerides a type of fat in your bloodstream or obesity, which associated with insulin resistance and insulin resistance is when your fat, blood sugar is not circulate round the cell as use to be and your blood sugar become high.

Age
The elderly people have a great risk of develop prediabetes and age from 45-50 of age have increased risk of develop type 2 diabetes and for children under age has also develop type 1 diabetes.

Prevention of type 1 diabetes

Type 1 diabetes mostly is cause by an autoimmune condition, but at this moment the cause is unknowing and in the other hand there are no way to prevent type 1 diabetes to occurring an meanwhile others researchers also emphasis that a trial shown some evidence of risk reduction that people who have other type of diabetes can be prevented or delay the development of diabetes complication by keeping their blood sugar level in target range and with the help of medical check-up insulin injection, the early sign and symptoms can be detect to prevent complication.

What Is Type 2 Diabetes

Type 2 diabetes is a process where by your pancreas cells do not make enough insulin to the bodies to be use as energy, called glucose (sugar), because the little insulin that your body produced is not work correctly in the body (known as insulin resistance). At the time of circulation the key mange to unlocking the cells for insulin to circulate round, but not enough for glucose to serve as energy to the body and them the glucose start accumulate and build up in the blood stream. During the circulation your blood glucose builds up to become higher than normal levels in the body and then your blood glucose become high that you can't control it, them your glucose rise to high level and type 2 diabetes was formerly known as non-insulin-dependent and type 2 diabetes is very common in young adults, teens and children known as roughly 90% of all diabetes cases in worldwide. We don't know what mechanism that cause type 2 diabetes disorders, but understanding genetic predisposition usually present and this could be a family history of the illness and other condition triggered by lifestyles, overweight or obesity factors. In a new research said that people with type 2 diabetes usually appears from over the age of 40-50 year of age, because type 2 diabetes is the common form of disorder in worldwide and it cause by different factors including insulin resistant, a condition whereby muscle, liver and fat don't produce enough insulin for body to be used. Type 2 diabetes can be manifested in the middle age and special older people are at risk of develop type 2 diabetes, but genetic dispositioned, overweight, poor diet and environmental factors are known as the most seriously trigger of type 2 diabetes. Type 2 diabetes also occurs when the hormone insulin is not used effectively by the cells in your body and insulin is needed for cells to take in sugar (glucose) from the bloodstream and convert it into energy use.

Prognosis of Type 2 Diabetes

When you are diagnose of type 2 diabetes in your early 40's means five to ten years off your average life expectancy shorter than normal population without diabetes and however with the new advance treatment and improvement of technology on recent years with diabetes association help to reduce life expectancy. Especially people with type 2 normally suffering of heart disease and which is known as the leading cause of death over the years and type 2 sufferers should follow up with healthcare team and GP recommended medication regime that would help to minimises the risk of long-term complication.

The cause and risk factors of type 2

Fami type 2 develops when your body become resistant to insulin that pancreas produces or when is unable to provide enough insulin, although genetic predisposition, lifestyle and environmental factors can cause the onset of diabetes disorder and with the combination of many factors can cause your body insulin resistance when your body doesn't use the insulin correctly, because insulin is a naturally hormones produce by pancreas and it release it when we eat any type of food and insulin help circulate it round the bloodstream into the cell were is use as energy. There are genetic predisposition, obesity, environmental trigger and geographical factor which increase the risk of insulin resistance. In other way round the cause and risk factors for type 2 diabetes is unclear, because the new researchers don't fully emphasis why some people develop prediabetes or type 2 diabetes and it's clear that a certain factors increase the risk of develops diabetes, including the follow are.

Genetic Factors
Family members who have been diagnosed with diabetes type 2 are at a higher risk of develop this disease and

your risk increases if a parent or sibling has type 1 and 2 diabetes in the family.

Diet

Eating unhealthy foods that contain more fat content, less fibre tends to cause type 2 diabetes.

Weight.

The more fatty tissue you have, the more resistant cell insulin and inactivity or less active you are also at risk to develop diabetes and with daily physical activity help control your weight loss and help to circulate your blood cells all round your bodies.

Race

Although it's unclear why people of certain races, including African, African American, Indians and Asian are at higher risk of develop diabetes.

Age

Your risk increases as you getting older and this may be because you tend to do less exercise, lose muscle mass and gain weight as you age is going along, but type 2 diabetes is also increasing dramatically among adolescents, children, and younger adults of ages.

How serious is type 2 diabetes

Type 2 diabetes is a serious medical condition that often requires the use of anti-diabetic medication, or insulin to keep blood sugar levels under control and however the development of type 2 diabetes and its side effects, complications can be prevented if detected and treated at an early stage. Prediabetes or metabolic disorder, type 2 diabetes can potentially be avoided through diet lifestyle change and regular exercise. According to the International Diabetes Federation (IDF), more than 371 million people across the globe have diabetes disease and this figure is also account for predicted to rise to over (550 million by 2030) and the total global diabetes rate is 90% are living with type 2 diabetes, but it was estimated that up to half of these people are unaware of their condition (undiagnosed diabetes) and in the UK, more than 2.7 million people has been diagnosed with type 2 diabetes and furthermore 750,000 people are believed to have the symptoms, but not yet to be diagnosed.

Prevention of type 2 diabetes

Type 2 is the most common type of diabetes and meanwhile prevention is the major things you can do to prevent the onset of diabetes as first priority if you are at risk of develop type 2 diabetes, such as overweight or you have a family history of the disease. Diabetes prevention is as base on what you eat every day, more physically active, healthier foods and losing a few weight is great prevention of onset diabetes and it's never too late to start managing your lifestyles, manage a few changes in your lifestyle it might help you avoid the serious health complications of diabetes, such as heart disease, nerve and kidney problem. Although with good effective treatment of diabetes mellitus can reduce the onset of long-term complication of type 2 diabetes, because so many people with type 2 has develop Microvascular and Macrovascular complication by the time their condition been diagnose and the following is prevent type 2 diabetes.

Healthy weight
Being overweight BMI who is greater than 27 that contributed to developing type 2 diabetes and if you are overweight you should look at other way to reduce your weight by 6% to 10% of your body and to reduce this you should cult down your portions of food and being daily physical active.

To reduce food portion
Choose healthier food and to cut off portion is the best way to reducing and limit sugary food and the best is to choose whole grain, vegetable and dairy products and be

advised to take everything in moderate and limit your alcohol intake and eat well balance meal to spread throughout the day to keep your blood glucose level in healthy balance.

Exercise
Exercise is very essential to the body to help circulate your insulin, blood glucose and also help to prevent type 2 diabetes is to lose weight if you are insulin resistant and this may also improve your blood pressure and cholesterol. Exercise keeps jour heart rate normal and sleeps better with the help of 30 minute exercise a day or 150 minute a week to keep you healthy.

Check your risk of diabetes
You need to take risk assessment test and known more about your onset of developing type 2 diabetes in early stage and if your score is A 12+ this indicates that you are at great danger and may be your doctor will referred for lifestyle modification program that can helps you reduce your risk of type 2 diabetes.

Your weight management
Why overweight or body fat abdomen can increase the body's resistance to the hormone insulin in your blood stream and it can lead to type 2 diabetes.

Limit your alcohol drinking
Drinking too much alcohol can result of weight gain or it's may increase your blood pressure and triglyceride range levels, especially men should follow up a recommended unit per day not more than two standard drinks a day and for women should have no more than one unit a day.

Quit smoking
Smoking is the biggest risk of developing type 2 diabetes than non-smokers in wide world..

Reduce your risk of cardiovascular disease
This is a good advice because any diabetes and cardiovascular disease have so many risk factors that cause complication to your body, including obesity and physical inactivity to do things.

Regular check-ups
The more you get older, it's important for you to check a regularly, your blood glucose, blood pressure and blood cholesterol range.

The Difference Between Type 1 and Type 2 Diabetes

There are two most important types of diabetes, type 1 diabetes and type 2 diabetes which has several differences from each other's, example the cause, symptoms, management and characteristic. This is also referred to who diabetes is affected and what effect does it has on the human body and there are others way to analysis the difference between the two similarities and the comparison on both section is as follow.

What Causes Diabetes Type 1 and Type 2

The cause of type 1 diabetes is unknow due to family history and is also occurs when the immune system, who fighting infection attacks and destroys the insulin that producing beta cells from the pancreas and in other way round a type 1 diabetes is also caused by genes and environmental factors, such as viruses, that might contributed to the disease which reducing the body's ability to produce sufficient insulin to regulate and circulate the blood glucose levels into the bloodstream as energy use. At the time insulin is not produced at all or is produced insufficient amounts of glucose for body to be use.

Type 2 diabetes is a condition whereby the body does not produce sufficient insulin, but it does supply insulin, not enough for body to use as energy and later the body's cells become resistant to the effects of insulin. This results in which build-up of glucose in the blood stream when cells has been starved of energy supply for very long time and this condition continue persistently in high glucose levels it will damage the blood cell. The used of insulin in body is not only to prevent hyperglycaemic emergencies, but is a safeguard that helps to prevent long-term complications of diabetes by correcting fasting level. Here are some different cause between type1 and types 2 diabetes, include different stages of disease which emphasis how extra insulin is not required, but to some people that does not require exogenous insulin for blood glucose control to survive. There are also numerous medical concerns of determinedly high levels of blood glucose in your body and the most serious one that onset the complication of kidney failure, eye problems (blindness), neurological damage and increased risk of cardiovascular problems like stroke and heart attack. Here are some of the cause of diabetes.

Genetic basis
In case of type 1 diabetes, the patients usually inherit from both parents as part of risk factors and while other factors can like infection, autoimmune system and medication can also cause type 1 diabetes and while type 2 diabetes has a generic factor that link to family history.

Climate/environmental
This can also trigger the onset of diabetes related to cold weather and while specially type 1 diabetes start to develop more often in winter than summer and this is more common in places of cold climates. According to the research type 2 diabetes sufferer is more common in people with low levels of vitamin D which will get from sunlight shine and vitamin

D are supports of immune to be function well with insulin sensitivity, this meaning that people living at cold winter atmosphere may face a higher risk of develop diabetes series than the people in tropical geographical climate. Diet Children who are born and following early diet may also play a huge role of develop type 1 diabetes according to a research and this is a common with people who were also breastfed and for those who first ate solid foods in early stage has develop diabetes at later ages or life.

The main symptoms of diabetes

In type 1 diabetes symptoms happen suddenly and can be life threatening for anyone who have onset of diabetes, but it's usually diagnosed quickly by your GP and the symptoms develop very promptly within over a few weeks in term and the symptoms main rapidly relieved once the diabetes is treated with recommendation or prescription of medication. In type 2 diabetes the symptoms may not be show rapidly and soon the condition start to develop gently over a period of years, the sign may only be picked up in a routine blood test immediately and the symptoms also relieved once diabetes is treated or under control. Before the symptoms appear or noticed a complications of diabetes may present in your system and for some reason diabetes symptoms can occur because all the food consuming, like carbohydrate which met to be converted into glucose to circulated insulin as energy through your bloodstream. Because at this time blood glucose is already build up in your blood cell and the exocrine work hard to reduce blood glucose levels and flushing the excess glucose out of the bloodstream through your kidney gland otherwise your start to experience sign and symptoms of diabetes include as following

Increase in urination
Higher glucose levels in your cell will now Flush the fluids in cell out frequently and this will increases the amount of fluid sent to the kidneys to secrete or urinate every time to time especially in the night time and make your body dehydrated.

Thirst
If you are a diabetes person your body start to dehydrated and you will become increase in thirsty drinking, because the symptoms of diabetes make you more thirsty and the more you thirst or urinate, the more you need to drink.

Fatigue
Feeling worn down or tire which is another common symptom of diabetes sufferer and you know glucose is one of the main bodies sources of energy supply and once the cells cannot absorb sugar into your body, you can become exhausted at any moment.

Hunger
Your body converts the food you eat into glucose that your cells use for energy and your cells need insulin to bring the glucose in order for you to gain more energy and at that time your body doesn't make enough insulin your cells struggle to use the little insulin your body produce to rich the target range.

Blurred vision
With short term, high glucose levels in the bloodstream can lead to cause swelling lens in the eye optical and this can also cause blurry vision to your eye site and with good control of your blood sugar which help to correct vision problems. Advised if blood sugar levels remain high for a very long time in your system that lead to total blindness if you are a diabetic person for life time.

Recurring infection
Your high blood glucose levels may make it harder for your body to heal from any injury and injuries like cuts, sores stay open longer than normal and this can lead to develop infection immediately. In some cases many people don't notice that they have high blood sugar levels on your system, because they don't feel or sensitivity at all and the elevation of blood sugar raise, then you begin to experience long-term complication, such as

Weight loss
Weight loss also fall under the categories of the sign and symptoms of diabetes and when you start losing glucose through regular urination from you also lose A lot of calories and fatty in your body. In a process of this your diabetes may keep the sugar from your food carbohydrate not getting circulating to destination cells that lead feeling hunger in your body. Weight loss will affect your body to be continue losing weight, especially people with type 1 diabetes. Excessive sugar in your bloodstream can lead to brain, nerve damage and during the time you may be experience or notice tingling and loss of sensation in your feet and hands, you may also notice burning pain in your arms, gum. Your diabetes disorder may weaken your ability to fight germs in your body, which can develop to increases the risk of infection in your gums and in your bones in between your teeth.

Dry mouth and itchy skin
Because you are been diagnose with diabetes your body has used all the fluids to make sure your body get moisture and because a diabetic patient away gets less moisturise or skin could get dehydrated, mouth may feel dry and genitals itchy from the skin and sexual remitted infection which can be repeatedly come back if you are

diagnose with type 2 diabetes or left untreated could be dangerous.

Slow healing sores or cuts
As a diabetes person you may experience complication any time or over time and your high blood sugar level can affect your glucose level in the body and that cause of nerve disruption makes it more harder for your healing wounds to heal quickly and with poor circulation could result in slower healing sore.

Nausea and vomiting
This happened when your body helps to burn fat and in this process your body build up ketones that build up in your bloodstream which can cause dangerous levels in your body or probably life-threatening condition called diabetic ketoacidosis in your body or urine (kidney) can lead to coma or death.

Dizziness
This is a common to individual, because several dizziness is a sign or symptoms of diabetes due to high or low level of blood glucose on your blood cell or also when you are dehydrated, because diabetes cause all kind of sign for many days or at lasting longer time, there are so many number causes to be investigated.

Gestational Diabetes

Gestational diabetes is a formed of short term condition that established during pregnancy time and if confirmed that you have gestational diabetes, this mean your glucose is higher than normal average reading and when you have higher blood sugar reading, it's important to get treated immediately, because it can cause you and your baby health problems. Gestational diabetes occurs during pregnancy time and usually gestational diabetes is a diseases of insulin resistance as type 2 diabetes resistant, because pregnancy increase your glucose or insulin to keep or reserved more insulin for growing baby and in some cases this usually happened during the second or third of pregnancy with women and some time it occur with women who don't have any sign of diabetes before. Shortly after giving birth it usually goes away, but in some women diabetes can lead to type 2 diabetes without change of life style and what happens is that during the pregnancy, the placenta produce hormones that help the baby to grow and develop and with this hormone can be block the action of the mother insulin to circulate to the bloodstream and if a woman developed gestational diabetes during pregnant, you at risk of developing prediabetes or type 2 diabetes and this happened after birth, baby weighing more than 10 pounds (5 kilograms at birth), you're also at risk of type 2 diabetes in the nearest future. Gestation diabetes happened because pregnant woman need extra insulin or needs two to 3 times insulin than as before and this time your body is unable to produce extra insulin to serve as energy to the baby and them body build up or manifests instantly insulin and after baby born your body return to normal stage then that person can live normal life, but depend on your life styles change.

Symptoms of gestational diabetes

Gestational diabetes normally started after the beginning of 12 weeks of your pregnancy and you may not notice any sign and symptoms, because it's usually diagnosed in a screening test before symptoms start to develop. If gestational diabetes isn't follow up on time, you may develop the onset of type 2 diabetes and most of these symptoms are really quite common if most of the women are pregnant, but not always the caused of gestational diabetes and also depend on family or genetic history. One of the symptoms is as follow.

- By increased thirst
- By feeling tired
- By passing urine more often
- By feeling dry mouth

Diagnosis of gestational diabetes

This can be done in your first antenatal appointment clinic and your midwife will ask or carried out some basic assessment if you at risk of develop gestational diabetes and this also base on your answers to the question, a test can be offered at later on to find out if you've about to developed gestation diabetes disorder or not.

Treatment of gestational diabetes

After you're have being diagnosed with gestational diabetes, your GP might refer you to antenatal or diabetes clinic were the doctors, midwifes, qualify nurses and dieticians who have gain experienced will look after your pregnant immediately. Your antenatal appointment will be more than women who don't have any gestational diabetes disorder, because any treatment carried out will help to keep your blood glucose low enough to help prevent your baby to be fully diabetes and you'll also need to test your BM day by days and more training, information leaf fleet paper would be given how to check your blood glucose level from time to time.

Self-help
You need some advice from your doctor or a dietitian how to manage gestational diabetes by chosen a changes to your lifestyle and your diet, how much exercise you can do and portion of food you want to take by doing this it may help keeping your blood glucose level to lower position and to reduce the risk of diabetes onset.

Eat a healthy balanced diet
This is one of the things that can help to keep your blood glucose level steady within the average range, include

eating enough carbohydrates that release energy slowly into your cell. One examples of these types of food includes oat, bread, cereals, wholegrain, pasta and sweet potatoes and onion are very important to keep active and some daily activity, exercise when you're pregnant, because this can help reduce your risk of developing gestational diabetes disorder or type 2 diabetes.

Medicines

Medication comes after you've tried all ways to reduce or control gestational diabetes by making a lifestyle changes, but if not do some daily exercise always, have a walk for once in a day or for two weeks long and if hasn't made any changes, then your GP or doctor need to prescribe a prescription medication to enable you to control your blood glucose level after birth. In other way round your doctor may put you on medication metformin which help to reduce your glucose level in the beginning.

Prevention of gestation diabetes

It's important for women to prevent gestational diabetes before get pregnant either to lose weight at first if you're overweight and start planning a regular physical activity and there are no guarantees when gestational it comes, but when you are pregnant eat more healthy food so that you can adopt a healthy habit of eating a good diets when pregnancy and when you develop gestational diabetes, these healthy choices of eating balance diets may also reduce your risk of having it in future pregnancies or developing type 2 diabetes in the nearest future. At the beginning of your pregnancy early parental care and regular visit healthcare centre helps to improve your health and wellbeing of your baby and a parental screening also stated at weeks 12-20 which help to detect you early develop gestational diabetes and preconception planning may help to prevent or reducing some threat that associate with gestation diabetes weight gain. There're other strategies that can use to reduce or improve insulin in your body which are

Maintaining a healthy weight

Weight control during or after birth is the biggest issues with people suffering of gestational diabetes and because being overweight you will be at risk of developing fully diabetes type 2 or to insulin resistance when you are pregnant. If you are overweight that doesn't mean you will have gestation diabetes during your pregnancy, because individual differences or you at risk of having gestational. Having a high blood glucose level, sometime it may be transferred to your baby, because your body it would be excessive growth of your baby when is born.

Exercise and Diabetes

If you're been diagnoses as gestational diabetes and as you were told by your GP you should know that diabetes and exercise work together, because physical activity comes in many way like dancing, gardening and yoga and daily activity also help to lower your blood glucose, cholesterol and enhance your mood degree level when you in relationship or with friends group.

Food and fitness

Healthy eating and physical activity are important to help to bring good outcomes of your blood sugar controls level and at least daily physical activity for 30 minute a day would help shape up the outcome of your gestational diabetes.

Fibre intake

Is better for pregnant women to increase fibre intake by 10 grams per day would be better to reduced risk of gestational diabetes when you are pregnant or you're planning to get pregnant by 30% and ten grams of fibre would be a cup of cooked or kidney beans and can be also take fibre supplements in a drugs store to help improve your glucose monitor.

The complications of gestation diabetes

A gestation diabetes can be manageable through your blood glucose levels during your pregnancy period and is also a tremendously to your health and unborn baby and in some women, gestational diabetes can be control with the help of lifestyle changes in diet and regular physical activity, but, especially in most cases, doctor can prescribe medications including insulin injecting if required to manage your prediabetes, but this happen after the birth of your baby. However, gestational diabetes that's not monitor well can cause problems for you and your baby in short time, because a qualify nurses, midwife and dietitians will help you reach your goal to set up a targets reading range for your blood glucose levels that will help reduce the risk of complications and to have healthy successfully pregnancy babies.

The Complications that may affect your baby

Excessive birth weight. Additional glucose in your bloodstream crosses around the placenta can causes you and your baby's pancreas to make you produce additional insulin in your blood cell and this will help your baby to grow too large size called (macrosomia).

Early birth and respiratory. A mother's who have developed high blood sugar might be at risk of early premature labour and delivering her baby before its due time and if you're suffering of gestational diabetes and your babies come early before due day might experience respiratory distress syndrome (called breathing difficult).

Low blood sugar called (hypoglycaemia). A mother of gestation diabetes, when their babies begins to start develops low blood sugar (hypoglycaemia) within a short period and severe episodes of hypoglycaemia may trigger seizures in the baby and later with the help of future monitor it will return the baby's blood sugar level to normal target range.

Type 2 diabetes later in life. According to new researcher who said that babies of mothers who have gestational diabetes have a higher risk of developing type 2 diabetes and obesity later in life.

High blood pressure. Gestational diabetes increases your risk of high blood pressure which can cause a serious complication of pregnancy that make you and baby lives threaten than any other condition.

Future diabetes. If you have being diagnose with gestational diabetes you have more likely to develop diabetes in later life and to prevent the onset of gestational diabetes, you need to choose a healthy lifestyle by eating healthy foods and do a regular exercise which can help reduce the risk of develop type 2 diabetes.

The cause of Gestational diabetes

During pregnancy the hormones in your body placenta can lead to a build-up of glucose in the bloodstream that can slab the effect of insulin that your body produce less efficient, because your pancreas that produced insulin can't no longer handle it, then the blood glucose become rise up which can cause gestational diabetes, also during pregnancy the pancreas produce and increase insulin double times the normal amount, but knowing you at risk of insulin resistance and other hand pregnancy places a heavy demand on insulin to the body and in some women they can overcome this resistance, but if glucose remains in the bloodstream and the levels begin to rise, which can lead to gestational diabetes.

Along with your pregnancy a lot of things happened, because your physical sign and the hormone your body produce it hard for the cell to use insulin in normal way as before and this will put yourself and baby at risk of insulin resistance, because in some women they can't produce enough insulin to meet the needs of your body. At this moment the causes of gestation diabetes during pregnancy cannot be over emphasis, because this base unknown fact that there are several number of risk factors that can increase the chances of develop gestational disorder through pregnancy, like, obese, family history and ethnicity, groups that in higher risk of gestational diabetes. Some of the risk factors for gestational diabetes are when a woman is pregnant which link to develop gestational diabetes, but some special women are at greater risk than others and the risk factors for gestational diabetes include.

Age
Women older than age 25 are greater high risk of develop gestation diabetes during pregnancy and family history can also increase the risk of develop gestation diabetes especially family with type 2 diabetes or sibling.

Weight
As diabetes patients and being overweight before pregnancy increases your risk of develop gestation diabetes.

Race
This can also referred to majority men and women who are black, Hispanic, American Indian or Asian are more likely to develop gestational diabetes during pregnancy time.

Human placental
These happen when hormone produced in the placenta that helps break down fat from the mother to provide.

Diabetes Management

Diabetes can be managed carefully watching out for some key point to be follow up and each individual that is recommended by NICE Guild and WHO stated that people who are suffering of diabetes should be undertake nine annual health checks, because it is so important that the people who are on treatment should follow up the nine health tests in regular occasion. High blood glucose should near to normal as possible 4–6mmol/l before meals and after meal is between 10 mmol/l or two hours after meal. The nine check health help patients to monitor and manage their condition to avoid complication issues and also help to reduce short and long-term complications such as heart disease, stroke and amputation. Diabetes can be also manageable by healthy eating, physical activity, losing excess weight, and medications and the other critical part of diabetes management is to reducing microvascular and macrovascular risk factors, like high blood pressure, high glucose levels, and smoking tobacco. The healthcare professional should educate patients the way to manage diabetes and self-care practices management which would benefit people with diabetes to stay healthier than ever. People who are been diagnose with type 1 diabetes need insulin dependent either by injection or an artificial pump to manage their swinging glucose level and this pump is a small device that you wear on your belt or your pocket and it deliver insulin 24 hours a day to the bloodstream and type 2 diabetes can also depend on medication to take control of high blood glucose level by following a healthy meal plan. Sometime serious type 2 diabetes also need insulin treatment or insulin dependent which can be recommended or use as high blood glucose monitor to reduce the risk of developing complication like eye, nerve, and kidney problem. Hypoglycaemia can happen when your glucose level is very lower than normal range and sometime this happened especially with elderly patients with poor control of diabetes disorder are vulnerable to develop a high risk of complication. The provision of self-management is to educate or training patients how to use self-management plan which is focusing on self-care behaviours, such as healthy eating, being active, yoga dance, take regular medications accordingly, learning a coping skills, and monitoring blood glucose level as recommended to overcome the appropriate balance of your cholesterol levels. To be fully manage your diabetes knowing your ABCs method which will help manage your blood pressure, cholesterol and glucose level and to achieved your goal toward your diabetes monitor to lower your risk of having heart attack or stroke by following the guideline and procedure accordingly. Why A for a1c test, B for Blood pressure, C for Cholesterol and S for Stop smoking and in recent research who also said that diabetes cannot be cure despite the fact of medication involvement, but can be manageable with your lifestyle changes which help to prevent the onset of long and short term diabetes complications and the goals of managing your diabetes disorder is as following.

Staying healthy

To stay healthy eating with all type of diabetes should make a choosing foods that is low in carbohydrates and vegetables, grains, fruit, beans and low-fat dairy products with little portion including diet weight control which would a beneficially to you and disorder. All type of diabetes need to eat healthy foods with the right balance meals a day and regular physical activities is the perfect recommendation with diabetes especially people taking two or more injections of insulin each day and with the help of family member or diabetes specialist, nurses will talk to you, explained how the procedure work and give you the necessary support for your needs.

Sugar intake

Sugar intake is known as carbohydrate which can be found in any foods naturally and sugar in fruit is also known as fructose and if you are type 1 diabetes and we all known that your pancreas is faulty and has been destroyed by immune system not only sugar intake can cause to have a type 1 diabetes mellitus and type 2 diabetes by consuming sugary drink and foods that can also cause fat that may contributed to your diabetes, or by consumed food more than what your body needs that can also lead to gain much weight from junked foods and most food contains some natural sugar (even carrots and potatoes) and it's possible to avoid it altogether would be better and eating foods that release sugar more slowly would be helpful. Some types of sugar, simple carbohydrates found in sweets, chocolate, or consuming sugary drinks and cakes will raise the blood sugar higher more quickly than others. By eating fruits contain natural sugar help to reduce your blood glucose and meanwhile alcohol intake or beer can also raise your blood sugar quite quickly than others, but if you are physically inactive or overweight the best way to manage your blood sugar is therefore to get yourself fit and let your body do the rest by naturally way.

Your Blood fats (lipids)

In recent research said that too much fat in the blood cell can contributed towards heart disease, stroke and blood fats include cholesterol and triglycerides are worst when you diabetes person and the level of triglyceride in the body should be less than 1.7mmol/l and while a cholesterol level not less than 4mmol/l. Anyway there is other way to decrease your blood cholesterol by doing some little exercise, eating low-fat diet food, and also participate on regularly activity or walk. If your GP seen your blood levels are still high, you might prescribe tablets to lower your weight gain and keeping your healthy body weight loss is vital to managing your diabetes and that will also help reduce your blood glucose levels down in other way round and gain your healthy lifestyle back, render than carrying more weight that will increases your risk of heart disease or stroke. Food Healthy eating is a keystone of living good weather you are without diabetes or not and you need to understand how foods affect your blood sugar levels. But your disorder will determine what type of food you eat or portion you consume at a time, but is also the combinations of food types you eat. The major key to many diabetes management plans is to education how much amount of carbohydrates you are be taken, because carbohydratcs are group of foods that often have the biggest effect on your blood sugar levels, because people taking mealtime insulin, it's crucial to know the amount of carbohydrates on your food, so that you can get the proper insulin dosage. It is important to know the portion size that is right for each type of food you ate, know the food you eat often and make a plan from the meals you enjoy, use measuring scale or cups so that the exact portion of carbohydrate is used.

Medication

The medication insulin and other diabetes is one that is use as a therapeutic way of lower your blood sugar levels when physical activity taking place or balancing your diet alone aren't enough for managing diabetes disorder, because the efficacy of these diabetes medications hangs on the timing and dosage taking daily and if you are also taken other medications for other condition can also upset your medication and your blood sugar levels become higher. Sometime people with type 2 diabetes can also achieve their target glucose levels with diet and exercise and some people still depended on diabetes tablet or insulin therapy in many occasionally and meanwhile doctor will make decision about what type of medication you would be on depend on your blood glucose level and any others medical condition you have, but insulin and metformin would be general first classes of drugs to be used for type1 and type 2 diabetes which help to control your blood glucose level in a several ways. If you have any issues taken diabetes medication should reported to your GP or contact whenever you experience any change to high level, the dosage may require adjustment if the medication may upset your blood sugar levels and especially liquid medications mix with sweet sugar to sweeten up the taste must be reported immediately.

Illness

What happened when you're sick, your body produces more stress, linked with hormones that help your body, fight the illness and during your illness would also raise your blood sugar level and especially when you have an infection and temperature goes high, your body produces less responded to insulin you injecting in your bloodstream. Being sick your body also produce more glucose and your glucose level is rise up, because you are eating less and you can also produce ketones when you are sick, because your body is unable to use glucose as energy, because of your insulin injections and not properly working as well your time of illness ketones remained or store in the bloodstream will turned or lead to diabetic complication called ketoacidosis (DKA) which can someone end up in coma and to manage you illness when you are diabetes keep your blood glucose in other just near target range to prevent the development of ketones or ketoacidosis in your blood cell.

During your brief illness you need to open your appetite and force yourselves to eat more food to help you recovery an time and however, if you're unable to eat because of nausea or vomiting, talk to your local doctor and some case you may need to amend your insulin dose or stop taking your medication because of the complication of hypoglycaemia. Whenever you're sick drink lots of water or other fluids that don't add calories, such as tea, that will enable you stay hydrated.

Alcohol Advice

If you're suffering of diabetes you use insulin or some other medication you're more likely to have a hypoglycaemia at the long run, because alcohol drinking it's reduce your body ability to recover when your blood glucose level are falling, because your liver store or reserved glucose which can be release back into the bloodstream. When body needed it and sometime your alcohol consumption stand on the way of your liver to have a good ability to function effectively, because blood has been affected by alcohol intake and after drinking alcohol then your liver start busy with full of metabolising and within a short time your blood sugar level raise. To utilised your alcohol or medication intake at the same time is quite difficult and drinking alcohol can also result in lower your blood sugar level down. Alcohol intake can complicate diabetes sugar level, such as nerve damage and eye disease and while alcohol intake is recommended for diabetes patients not to drink more than one unit per day for women of any age and for men over 60 years older. Advised after drinking, check your blood sugar level before you go to bed, because it can lower your blood sugar levels for long time and if your blood sugar isn't between 5.6 and 7.8 mmol/L) or is lower than normal, have a snack before go to bed to hostage your blood sugar level.
Drinking alcohol has many effects on an individual with or without diabetes and even a small unit alcohol can be dramatically increase your blood glucose levels on your system, because alcohol contains many calories and too much consumption can be so difficult to manage your diabetes, while alcohol intake also increase triglyceride and cholesterol level on your system.

Stress

If you're emotional stressed, your body hormones will produces and response to prolonged stress and during this time your blood sugar level may be rise to high level. To take control of yourself, when you're stress that would affects your blood sugar level, but you need to fight back by using relaxation techniques to avoid common stressors and begging to practice physical exercise that would help relieve your stress and lower your blood sugar level. By using a new coping strategies for stress mechanism and you will also discover that working with a psychologist or clinical specialist worker can also help you identify your stressors mechanism. Stress can be a challenge to deal with diabetes management especially type 1 diabetes and coping with it is a seriously issues because of the serious effect it can have on your daily health and diabetes and stress is a physical and emotional reaction to difficult situations that can elevate your blood glucose level.

What happened to people who aren't diabetic person which they have compensatory mechanisms to keep blood glucose swinging out of control and the people suffering with diabetes, those mechanisms are either absent in insulin resistant, because they can't keep their blood sugar in place or control.

Diabetes and healthy eating

You need to eat good variety of nutritious food and healthy foods in your diet plan that will promote your healthy lifestyles and you also need to avoid snack food that contain sugary. Eating healthy foods can help control your high blood glucose down and cholesterol levels to be balance, also your blood pressure. This would be include a different selection of foods include foods high in fibre and low in fat would help reduce your glucose level and little salt intake will help promote your wellbeing calcium level and get fibre that helps to reduce cholesterol and

Triglycerides which help in your strengthens walls and it also contribute to helps your weight loss, management of blood sugar levels and help to prevent insulin resistance related to diabetes disorder people.

Healthy fish, eating fish at least twice a week and fish can be a good alternative to high-fat meats and some example, tuna and halibut have less total saturated fat and fish such as salmon, mackerel, tuna, sardines and bluefish are rich in omega-3 fatty acids, which promote heart health by lowering blood fats called triglycerides, cholesterol in your body. When you are diabetes person daily nutrition and physical performance are vital part of your healthy lifestyle which can help improve your diabetes diet plan and along side with other profits by following your healthy meal plan to improve your glucose target range and is also vital to take your medication if you are taken meds to keep your recommendation goal by healthcare professional.

Diabetes meal plans

Diabetes meal plan for weight loss is known as a simple eating plan that promotes consumption of different varieties of food or fruit and healthy nutritious and diabetes meal plan offers specific food that help to control blood sugar level, food that contained diet balance that will help your blood glucose levels in safer range. The must essential task if you are diagnosis with diabetes or prediabetes, follow up the diabetes meal plan and protocol so that you can meet your target goal easy or straight away by bringing little healthy adjustments to your eating behaviours lifestyles.

A diabetes meal plan is about what, when and how much to consume to get the nutrition you need in your body as a diabetes patients that can keep your blood sugar levels in your target range and you'll want to plan for a steady, secure meals to avoid high or low blood sugar levels. Some time eating carbs can raise your blood sugar level faster and higher than protein or fat you are expected and eating fibre can also help you manage your blood sugar level, like sweet potatoes, won't raise your blood glucose level as other carbs with little or no fibre.

Weight Loss

Weight lose is the most important decision you're ever make to help manage your diabetes disorder and lose a small amount of weight as you plan will help and also reduce the risk of heart diseases, stroke and some of other diseases.

Eating healthy food choices is very important when someone battling with diabetes as excess calories and fat-rich diets start to build up in a higher blood sugar levels in the body and if left unchecked for long time, the high blood sugar can cause health problem, especially heart and kidney impairment. A diabetes meal plan is not only to provide an effective on your blood glucose and also to keep you blood sugar level to normal range for a healthy weight loss. Diabetes meal plan for weight loss is a simple eating plan that promotes consumption of different varieties of food or fruit diets in practical numbers of mealtimes and healthy nutritious diabetes meal plan offers specific food items that help you control blood sugar levels. What matter is to balance your blood glucose levels in safer range is much essential task, if you are one of the diabetes or prediabetes patients.

Sleeping patterns

According to new research who said that sleeping patterns both short and long hour sleep daily also contribute to higher risk of developing type 2 diabetes and while a short sleep may impair the balance of hormones regulating food intake and also trouble with energy balance. People with diabetes who having long sleep durations may be a sign of sleeping disorder and this happen if you are obesity and that mean have obstructive sleep apnoea syndrome. The sleep schedule is one of the most important rhythms in the human body and our body needs from six to 8 hours of sleep every day in order to repair itself and refresh itself for the next 24 hours duty and it may be necessary for us to change sleeping habits pattern. Whether temporarily or permanently as long as you take the time to understand your sleeping habits and you can learn how to adjust your sleep schedule on time.

People who are diabetes, sleeping pattern can disturb your blood glucose levels and glucose control can also be affected in area of trouble sleeping pattern, because is had getting a special good night sleep and insomnia can also a big roots in blood glucose control level and which are the key role to your heathy sleep pattern. Lack of sleep pattern can alter your hormone in balance which can be affected your food intake and weight gain from any food you are eating. Having a diabetes is a huge challenging in any circle by eating an excess amount of food to gain much energy through the consumption of calories and this can cause you your blood glucose levels to rise any moment and it had to achieve attired amount of good sleep and this may result you having these same sleepless night situation.

Healthy carbohydrates

Carbohydrate foods play a vital role in our diet today and also offer the best energy source to the body as glucose to the blood cell, especially to the brain. What insulin does in the body is to takes the glucose away and converted it from carbohydrate produces out to circulate into the muscles, liver and use as energy to the body. The carbohydrate food are very good sources of fibre, because healthier carbohydrates food such as minerals, vitamins, fruit, vegetable, bean, peas are help to low-fat dairy products to maintained your body and help for your bowels. All food type or carbohydrate you eat are used to broken down into glucose in the bloodstream and the body supplied insulin automatically to resettle the glucose that enters the body from the food carbohydrate down, because as an diabetes patient your body doesn't produce any insulin to the blood cell then you need insulin or pump to support yourself and lower your glucose level in your blood cell, after eating some setting food called carbohydrate foods and some carbohydrate can cause your blood sugar to be higher than normal range.

Fibre rich foods
The food that is high in **fibre** are known to lower blood cholesterol and blood glucose levels like grains, oats and other high **fibre foods** should be added in your diabetics foods, noodles, pasta should be avoided in your daily recipe food.
Dietary fibre includes all parts of plant foods that your body can't digest or absorb easily and fibre moderates how your body digests you food and helps control blood sugar levels. Foods that are high in fibre include vegetables, fruits, nuts, legumes, peanut (beans, peas and lentils) wheat brain help to reduce your risk of getting diabetes by improving your weight control and blood sugar level.

Good fats

The type of good fat food found in our food quite saturated and the saturated fats is known as fat that present in higher amount from animal product, like meat and cheese which increase bad cholesterol in the body that build up a fatty material in the artery walls. While unsaturated fats food is a fats found in fish, olive oil, nuts and other foods process introduce good cholesterol that help lower your levels of glucose level and also lower you blood pressure by eating fruit called, avocados, pecans, walnuts, olives and peanut oils, but don't overdose it, because all fats are high in calories. If you are a diabetes patients get more physical activity because is very essential when control you glucose level and is also a key part of managing diabetes along with proper meal planning.

Avoid fad diets

Eating low-carb diets or other fad diets may help losing more weight at the beginning of your diabetes program and their effectiveness is also use to preventing the onset of diabetes complication, by strictly limit a particular food group to be eating to keep maintaining your diabetes in under control.

As a diabetes patient using semi-skimmed milk is also recommended to improve your wellbeing and other low-fat dairy products, like grilling, steaming or baking foods is healthier than frying oil food, because all fats intake contain a lot of amounts of calories, so is advisable to limit your fat intake if you are planning to lose weight regarding to your diabetes disorder. Loss extra weight if you're overweight, diabetes prevention may be depend on how you weight balance and every weight loss mater especially when you are diabetes that can improve your health life and regular exercised also reduced the risk of developing prediabetes to type 2 diabetes. Overweight and weight is a common recommendation for the treatment for type 2 diabetes.

Eat plenty of beans

A research found out that eating beans is recommended as one of the best diabetics super food and the American Diabetes Association and Diabetes UK advises people with diabetes to add more beans into their daily food or no-sodium beans to several meals each week, because they are low in glycaemic and can help manage your blood sugar levels to target normal range. The beans also have protein and strong fibre as nutritional component to every meal and when planning your everyday meals remember that 1/3 cup of cooked beans is considered as one of the best diabetic food and one unit of beans provides about 70 calories and that is about 15 grams of carbohydrates consumption a day.

Foods to avoid

When you are diabetes patients, you are at risk of heart disease and stroke by increase the development of arteries blockage and to avoid this you can only allowed eat foods that containing the following group that would help you work beside your goal of a heart-healthy diet. The food that high-fat dairy products like animal proteins beef, hot dogs, sausage should be avoid and limit your daily calories from saturated fat and not more than 8 percent daily consumption and don't eat too many types of fats that are found in processed of snacks, shortening and stick margarines.

Self-Diabetes monitoring

Self-monitoring blood glucose mean you check your blood glucose level by yourself at home or any were to identify your reading level whether is higher or lower and Self-monitoring of blood glucose (SMBG) is an important component of modern treatment for people with diabetes mellitus. When you are diabetes patient to manage your blood glucose is a way of avoid short and long-term of diabetes complications and self glucose monitoring is another way for you to take charge of your health, eating, being active has recommended for people with diabetes and health care professionals in order to achieve a successfully glycaemic control level and also to prevent hyper and hypoglycaemia.

Using a blood glucose meter that indicate the level of your glucose at that moment and it also tell you the correct effect of what type of food you eat after 2 hours before your glucose was taken and it's vital because glucose levels are always shifting during the day and evening/night time and so many things can trigger your sugar level to be high either food, or daily activity. A diabetes person may find self-monitoring as problematic for many reasons and for patient that carry materials glucose matter and prick themselves several times per day is frustrated with unpredicted results specially with l type 1 diabetes and also people with type 1 should be well educated and offer a structure to ensure they have the knowledge and skills to enable inject insulin according to carbohydrate intake to get the right dose. The goal of SMBG is to collect detailed information about level of blood glucose at four time a day and this will enable patients to maintained of a more continuous glucose level by more routines.

Risk Factors Leading To Diabetes

Many factors can contributed to increase the risk of the developing diabetes which can be happen especially in elderly people from above 50 year of age and diabetes sufferer is not only focus on who you are, because it can affected anyone on any age group, but can't be transfer" from one person to another or either in sexual relationship. Sometime most people who are diagnoses with type 2 diabetes have no sign and symptoms experience at all, it come on slowly, usually happened over the age of 40 plus and some time it might be up to ten years before you experience the sign and symptoms, but you can't change the risk factor behind diabetes disorder such as family history, Age or ethnicity or to prevent this you can change your lifestyle to make it better life, render than eating, gain weight or unphysical activity which can contributed to developing type 2 diabetes and change of life style can help delayed your chance of having type 2 diabetes in life. Diabetes risk factor also base on two different type of risk which are **Modifiable and Non-modifiable.**

Modifiable risk of diabetes can make healthy changes over night so that you can reduce risk for diabetes or delay its development progression and changes can also improve your overall quality of your daily life and some of the risk factor are Obesity, Physical activity, cholesterol, high blood pressure, smoking which you can manage to change and get a better life.

The risk are Obesity

Obesity is the major cause of type 2 diabetes to some people and this has contributed a huge risk factors to develop type 2 diabetes and in worldwide millions of people that develop type 2 throughout are facing obesity disorder which know as number one of the risk factor to diabetes. In the UK many adults and children are recorded as number one obesity lead to diabetes and other hand a numbers of people who suffering of obese continue to climb up by percentage per year, the number of children being diagnosed with type 2 diabetes caused by obesity is much high in worldwide today and even in the UK. According to a new research who said that about one in three children are classed as obese disorder and 90 percent of people diagnose with type 2 diabetes each are overweight issues.

Physical activity

Daily physical exercise is very essential part of your diabetes management plan, because during your exercise, your muscles use sugar (glucose) for energy supply and while regular physical activity helps your body to utilised or circulate insulin more efficiently and also helps to lower your blood sugar level. The more active you work out, the longer the effect lasts for a long time. For example, the light daily activities like housework, gardening or being on your feet for long periods of walk can improve your blood sugar level. You are advised to check your blood sugar level before and after physical exercise, especially if you are taken insulin or medications that lower blood sugar to known the effectiveness of medication you are. Every day exercise help lower your blood sugar levels, especially if you're exercising for long distance and during your exercise if you are experiencing or aware of warning signs of low blood sugar in your body, such as feeling shaky, weak, tired, hungry, lightheaded, irritable, anxious or confused you should tell someone. However, before you start doing exercise drink plenty of water or other fluids to avoid dehydration that can increase your blood sugar levels and you also need to have a small snack or glucose tablet with you in case your blood sugar drops too low level and if you are planning to do exercise need at least 30 minutes of moderate physical activity in a day make it better.

High cholesterol

Too much fatty or poor cholesterol shape in your body can increases risk of developing diabetes and there is average numbers which your GP or doctor considered to be high cholesterol, HDL cholesterol ("good" cholesterol) levels of 35 or lower and triglyceride levels of 250 is consider to be higher. What is HbA1c level, the HbA1c and A1c has been recommended to show how well their diabetes is being controlled called Haemoglobin test, which is used to control or detect how is your diabetes blood glucose level over the past two to three months follow up reading. This measure has been used to know whether the recommended treatment of your diabetes is working well or not and if you've already been diagnosed with diabetes is obvious that you should do HbA1c test and this test to be done twice in year especially when you are on medication. Being diagnose your blood glucose tolerance test (GTT) can be also carried out any time without require a preparation, such as fasting test according to WHO suggested that HbA1c test could also be used to help diagnose type 2 diabetes with people who didn't known they got type diabetes initial. Diagnosed of diabetes is base an HbA1c result, if greater than or equal to 6.5% Result A1C Normal less than 5.7% Prediabetes 5.7% to 8.4% Diabetes 8.5% or higher Ideal levels blood glucose 6–8mmol/l before meals and up to 10mmol/l two hours after meals, Normal blood pressure with diabetes patients is 140/80mmHg, blood fats triglyceride level less than 1.8mmol/l total cholesterol less than 7mmol/l HbA1c 6.5% or below expectation 7.5% or below for those at risk of severe hypoglycaemia).

Your Blood pressure monitor

If you have been diagnose with diabetes your blood pressure should be checked by professional healthcare annually, because is very important as part of your diabetes health checked monitor and when your blood pressure is high, is called Hypertension and if continue you need treatment to bring it to normal level.

Blood pressure can put you at risk of developing all diabetes complications at place and with good recommendation of blood pressure levels control it will help you reducing the risk of heart disease and stroke. Blood pressure should be measured bellow 140/80 mmHg level when you are diabetes person or less. There are still other ways to help reduce your blood pressure by reducing your weight, eating less or low diet fat food, low salt intake and regularly physical exercises. However, in some cases if your blood pressure is still at risk or in high position then you most consults your GP or doctor to review your medication to avoid complication.

Smoking
Smoking is one of the greatest rough lifestyle that can contribute to risk factor to developing diabetes complications in life and what smoking does to the body as diabetes person it will affected all your circulation of blood by increasing your blood pressure and heart rate. This can cause complication to your small blood vessels narrower called microvascular disease and it's allows bad fatty material to build up in the wall vessel which can lead to heart attack, stroke and while other blood vessel called macrovascular disease can also interval and people diagnose as diabetes who found to be smoker has higher blood glucose levels ever. Smoking is known as addicted habit which can increase the risk of developing other many serious disorder which can be a life threating and damage to large blood vessels like cancer, Strokes heart attack and lead to poor glucose circulation into your bloodstream. The people who are not diabetes and never smoked should not start thinking about it or stop smoking, because smoking is really dangerous to people health especially people who are suffering of diabetes

disorder, because smoking bring the risk to developing blood vessel damage and naves complication.

Non-Modifiable risk factor which base on a number of element that surrounding the increasement of disorder, like prediabetes which lead to fully type 2 diabetes and is one of the characteristics of non-modifiable which referred to family history, genetic, age, ethnic and history of gestational diabetes. These condition can't be change due to exiting life history and is part of the risk that contributed to the development of diabetes and can be also prevented to reduce the onset of diabetes disorder and there few factors which are,

Family History

Family history is vital risk of developing diabetes and many other number of chronic disease can also lead from family genetic aspect and although you can't change family history and it is very vital for you to let your doctor to know if any diseases runs in your family. Example, diabetes status record also show that most people who has been diagnosis with type 2 diabetes have a family back ground disorder, such as brother, sister, sibling or suddenly history of type 2 in the family which played a long role as risk factor to others diseases. If you have family history of diabetes you are at risk, but these day if you have family member of diabetes, there are other way to prevent the onset of developing diabetes by lower the risk of having it. For example if you are overweight, try to loss weight immediately or do some exercise 30 minutes a day and make sure your healthy food choices will help you prevent or delay your type 2 disorder.

Genetic

Genetics diabetes play a huge role of developing both type 1 and type 2 diabetes in the family which have the high risk of developing disease disorder and in some family children more likely to develop type 1 and type 2 diabetes which based on genetic predisposition and others lifestyle could influence the child likelihood. The environment factors can also lead to developing of diabetes, because of predisposition factors which make some people vulnerable to diabetes disorder without knowing. In a recent event there are many way to reduce the risk of type 2 diabetes when you are aware of family history and taken a step to prevent the onset of diabetes and healthy lifestyle could prolong or lower the chance of developing diabetes by eating health food and being active to maintaining healthy weight. Grandfather, parents and children some time they all share similar chromosome and health issues regarding genetic aspect of diabetes, because the onset disease run in the family as inherited factors that can put you at risk.

Age

Your age is one of the biggest risk factors that also contributed to type 2 diabetes diseases, especially after 40 to 50 years of age, but you can't change your nature, but you can pan and work on other risk factors to reduce your risk of developing type 2 diabetes. According to others new research who said that the reasons while other ethnic groups has a higher risk of diabetes than others can't be overemphasis and but type in this picture is also increasing dramatically among the young and adolescent and type 2 diabetes started to rise up as you are getting older and it happened when people start to do less exercise, gain weight and loss of muscle mass from your body.

Diet

If you are eating a diet that is high in fat or calories your cholesterol will increases your risk of having diabetes, because is made of poor diet eating which can lead to obesity too and this will be another risk factor for diabetes sufferer. In another investigation also said the drinking cow milk in early stage or childhood of their life could cause of type 1 diabetes and a healthy diet that is high in fibre can also cause risk factor. Remember to watch out your portion size you eat at a time, because is very important and it might impaired your glucose tolerance (IGT) this is were by the level of blood glucose which is higher than normal in your bloodstream can cause complication.

By eating well will help control and reverse back your type 2 diabetes, because eating nutritional and physical activity are very vital part of a healthy lifestyle when you are being diagnosis with diabetes disorder and following up a meal plan can also keep your blood sugar in normal range.

COMPLICATIONS OF DIABETES

Diabetes complications are based on the negative parts of having the condition called diabetes milutus and there are a variety of problems that may develop with diabetes, but not every sufferer will develop or experience the same condition. Some of the complications are likely to happen if someone have high blood glucose levels or high blood pressure over a lengthy of time and taking good care of your blood glucose level, blood pressure daily is the best way to avoid complications of diabetes. Diabetes complication also referred to on short term and long-term condition which are divided into two divisions: **Macrovascular and Microvascular**, Microvascular is the distraction of the body organ that damage to small vessels in your body organs which formulated issues within the eye, foot, nerves and kidney problem. Meanwhile Macrovascular system is also a distraction of large blood vessel in the body that creating issues in large blood vessels, like cardiovascular, stroke and heart attack which lead to cause insufficiently of low flow blood to the leg. Long-term complications of diabetes is a serious disease if you are a diabetes patients and if not well managed it can lead to long-term complications which can affects many areas in your body. Diabetes complication can only build up gradually for years if not well manageable and the longer the person have diabetes, the higher the risk of complication to develop. The best thing is by keeping your blood sugar level, fat and blood pressure in control to normal range, together with healthy lifestyle, because this help avoid less risks of developing short and long-term condition.

Microvascular Complication of Diabetes,

Diabetic Retinopathy (eye disease) is the leading cause of blindness in worldwide and the cause leakage from the small blood vessels that supply the retina light-sensitive and vision at the back of the eye is defected. Keeping your blood pressure, glucose and fat levels under control will help to reduce the risk of developing retinopathy infection and it is suggested that people who are suffering from diabetes should have annually eyes screened check with specialist professional and there are camera equipment that can detect early retinopathy problem. Retinopathy means people with diabetes condition where by the blood vessels in the retina become damaged or destroy which lead to vision defect, because the retinopathy has several stages. As an diabetes person this happen at the early stages, but there are no sign and symptoms and suddenly you have only vision remitted and so having a full diabetes eye check or screening is essential to detect any early sign and early treatment would help to prevent more damages.

Macular oedema This is part of the retina that helps us to see things clearly and swelling up can happen when is affected area in retina blood vessel with plenty of fluid that build up within retina area causes vision blurry. Early intervention is better because this is when the lens of the eye becomes affected shoot pain and can cause vision to become inaccurate or sensitive to brightness. People with diabetes can develop cataracts at an earlier age of diabetes and with early intervention can be prevented the onset.

Glaucoma When your eye is affected by diabetes the pressure of the fluid within the eye builds up to a higher level than when is healthy and this pressure can damage the eye over time. The glaucoma can occurs in people with diabetes or not without diabetes people and but initially this more common in people with diabetes. The symptoms can be a daily patients complained of eye blurred vision and while in the other hand another symptom can also be appearing, because the most surrounding area is damage to the eyes, but in earlier stages there are some symptoms that may occur during and these need urgent intervention to reduce the level damage. If you are unfortunate to have flashes of light, blots and dots or you felt part of your vision is missing, seek urgent medical advice or contact optician specialist.

Nephropathy(kidney disease) Diabetic kidney disease can be happened by damage to small blood vessels which lead to nephrons failure and the diagnosis for small leakage levels of kidney disease can progress to proteinuria defects. In so many case the kidneys can be a failure any time and lead to dialysis or a kidney transplant. Kidney disease occurs when the kidneys start to fail to carried out the duty and the kidney disease start develops slowly to builds up glucose for a very long time, but is very important to detect it earlier stage and this condition it happened to people who have diabetes for over 15-20 years. But this condition is not rear and it happened 1-3 with diabetes patient in random, but with the help of recommended medication treatment and with early or good

Management would reduce the risk of develop kidney problem. Diagnosis on early warning sign can reduce the risk of develop urine protein and full routine blood test can carried out for kidney infection and early treatment stage can reduce the risk of kidney failure. The test can also carried out by control your high blood glucose, urine ketones ketoacidosis and high blood pressure regular.

Symptoms: Some case many patients have no symptoms experience, but the disease can be progress and they may experience tired, dizzy and even develop electrolyte imbalance in the body.

Diagnosis. On early warning sign and diagnosis can reduce the risk of develop urine protein and full routine blood test for kidney infection.

Treatment. Early stage of diagnosis can reduce the risk of kidney failure and this can be also carried out by control your high blood glucose and high blood pressure regular and also immediate intervention with doctor prescription of medication in early stage is better and to be followed up a dietician regime.

Neuropathy (nerve disease)
This is most common complication of diabetes which often affected the nerve system through different mechanisms and high blood glucose (hyperglycaemia) can cause or damage to the small blood vessel in the body nerves and decrease blood flow to the nerve system. As diabetes patient if nerve is damage this can lead to human loss of sensory feelings and can lead to impotence (sexual dysfunction) and is one of the common complication of diabetes that they all went through and if patients wound deterioration, because of slowly healing infection can lead to amputation. The high blood glucose levels in the bloodstream that will harm the blood vessels that transport oxygen and nutrients to the nerves. Note that people who drink large amounts of alcohol can also develop nerve impairment and while people who are lack of vitamin B12 deficiency can also develop a serious signs and symptoms of peripheral neuropathy to the body. Using long-term medication called metformin for diabetes for more than three to four years treatment can cause or raise your risk of lack vitamin B12 deficiency. To prevent nerve damage to your body is to keep your blood glucose levels in target range and if you are alcoholic person keep within the recommended guidelines and local Dr advice to prevent the onset of kidney disease or you are a heaving smoker stop smoking or if you don't smoke before, talk to your local doctor about any problems you have experience with your arms, feet, or legs, your stomach, bowels, or bladder.

There are different types of neuropathy disorder

Sensory neuropathy this is affected all area that carry messages from muscle, bones and skin to the brain and it is the common parts of neuropathy and mostly occurs in all over the body which lead to short site failure to sense area. Some symptoms include numbers of tingling and sensitivity to reach.

Autonomic neuropathy, this is where the area nerves is affected that control all round of the body and these include the sexual organs in both women and men (causing erectile dysfunction), intestine, sweat glands and the heart and some symptoms may vary depending on the part of the body that is affected.

Motor neuropathy, this is the parts area that involves in eyes and muscles of the legs and feet and sometimes is very painful, when cause muscle to be weak. This can lead to the development of foot defects or amputation.

Symptoms
Early warning sign can prevent human impotence and can decrease feet, nerves problem, which can be lead to a patient not recognise cuts, feeling pains and start to develop foot infection if not early intervention or treatment which can be lead to amputation of your body.

Diagnosis
Early diagnosis and sign can help for early recognition of the symptoms from health professional and these help patients to reduce the risk of develop impotence and amputation to the body.

Treatment
Early detection of the complication can help bring into blood glucose level under control and can be prevented or delay the onset of impotence.

Macrovascular Complications of Diabetes

Macrovascular Complications of Diabetes,
Macrovascular disease is defined as blood vessel disease, heart attack and stroke is the most dangerous disease that causes of death within the diabetes people and especially people with high cholesterol and high blood pressure levels medication which consider being one of the complications of diabetes. Referred to people who have been smoking for longer period of time and family history of cardiovascular disease, stroke are also contributed to high risk of diabetes complication and physical inactive also increase your risk of develop cardiovascular diseases of you are in a setting medication. Cardiovascular disease CVD (heart and stroke) this is also cause by hyperglycaemia that affected people with diabetes than the general population, because this is a common cause of early premature death for people with diabetes 1 and 2 type. The cardiovascular disease can lead to decrease blood flow or a blockage of arteries in the body that leading to heart attack, meanwhile if blood artery flows to the brain, it can cause a stroke immediately. To reduce the onset or your risk of complication you need to pick up any early sign warning and check your blood pressure at least twice in a week or more often if you have high blood pressure on top of your diabetes disorder or on medication. All diabetes patients need to have their HbA1c checked at least every six months or twice in a year to known the average glucose level within 6 month in a year and you can also have your cholesterol pathology tests such as an electrocardiogram (ECG) done or with daily exercise also be recommended from your local professional people.

Stroke, Diabetes is always goes with risk factor of a complication and it can cause physiology and pathology changes in your blood vessels and it will lead to cerebral vessels damage. A stroke happened when blood not reaches into your brain target and staved of oxygen supplied and nutrients, because the blood vessel who carry blood cell to the heart are damage due to too much glucose (sugar) in long period of time. So it better to keep your HbA1c level which can help prevent you blood vessel through your treatment regime and because the risk of stroke can be prevented.

Symptoms of early intervention warning sign can be varied specially chest pain to leg or without early intervention this could lead to confusion and paralysis and diagnosis of early warning sign and detection would delay the onset of complication of heart and stroke attack any time and also to prevent the risk factors of smoking habit, high blood pressure and high cholesterol or obesity would help stopping heart attack on expected situation. Stop smoking or reduce your weight is more essential to health treatment and control of your blood glucose monitor can delay the complication of cardiovascular disease. Strokes also fall into categories of heart attack in the brain and this happened when blood flow can't reach your heart and this obstruction can be occurred during a blood clot or break down in blood vessel to the function brain which can result death or stroke disability.

Diagnosis
Early intervention and detection of the complications can delay onset of progression to other level of heart attack and to learn how prevent the risk that can trigger the factors such as smoking, cholesterol, high blood pressure and obesity which can help reduce the complication.

Treatment
A good intervention and regular control of your blood pressure and stop smoking will help your risk factors with blood glucose monitor and medication treatment delay the cardiovascular complication of diabetes disorder.

Heart Disease
Heart disease is a complication issues that may affect people with diabetes if their condition is not under control for a long period of time and most it happened especially people suffering from type 1 and type 2 diabetes are more likely to be at high risk of heart attacks, strokes and high blood pressure continue to raise up more than normal target range. The coronary heart disease (CHD) or ischemic heart disease (IHD), is also contributed to reduction of blood flow to the heart muscle due to heaven blood pump or build-up in the arteries it will develop heart failure and which is the most common cardiovascular diseases including stable angina, myocardial infarction, and the immediate cardiac death.

The symptoms of cardiovascular disease may be individual different from others people and men are known to be likely to have chest pain and women are more likely to have the same symptoms along with discomfort chest pains and shortness of breath.

The cause of could be a complication of diabetes disorder and the damage to coronary arteries vessel or poor supply of nutrients and oxygen to the organ even high blood pressure that related to diabetes complication can also cause the onset of heart disease and obesity is another issues that can cause heart defect by having too much excess weight BMI index which can lead to develop cardiovascular condition in some diabetes patient..

Treatment, there are two major type of treatment which base on type 1 and type 2 diabetes complication and medications called beta-blocker treatment of heart failure and high blood pressure and surgery bypass to help correct the problem and other medication use to prevent blood clots of the heart.

Peripheral Disease
Peripheral is a potentially serious case which can develop in foot problem or start to manifest gradually if you are diabetes person, because of your nerve damage and blood vessel can stop the blood not to flow to the destination or to the vessels and if you are diabetes person it's important that you take your feet problems into a matter of concerns. As diabetes person, if your nerve damage in your feet or poor blood circulation to the feet, it will increases the risk of various foot complications and uncared of your poor wound, small sores or your breaks skin may turn into deep skin ulcers which mean can be gradually developed and once the skin ulcers get larger and larger or grow deeper you might develop foot ulcer as a result of amputation of the foot. To prevent peripheral, a patient should stop smoking immediately, because smoking narrow your blood vessels in your heart over a period of time and low flow blood to your heart especially to your lower limb. As a diabetes person a peripheral disease is a sign of blood fatty accumulation in the arteries condition called atherosclerosis and complication of diabetes which reducing blood flow to your heart, legs and brain that causes heart and stroke later in life.

Symptoms, can be vary to many people, but some people have the symptom of leg pain when taken a work, muscle pain, but it can be disappear any time and it can be from severity to mild discomfort moment to make it harder to walk or other physical activity.

Causes can be cause by deposit a fatty blood that builds up in the arteries vessel and reduce blood flow to wall that can affect the arteries through your body that supplying blood sugar to your limbs which cause peripheral arteries disease and the main cause is the blood vessel inflammation, injury to your limb which cause radiation to the muscles. Smoking and diabetes, Obesity and body mass index, High blood pressure and High cholesterol and family history or genetic predisposition can be the risk of peripheral disease.

Treatment of peripheral artery disease is based to reduce the onset of peripheral defect or change lifestyle to improve your mobility to prevent diabetes complication, medication and without treatment it will slow progress to high level of complication result in tissue damage or sore due to inadequate blood flow.

Atherosclerosis is a process in which blood, fats such as cholesterol and other substances build up on your artery walls. Eventually, deposits called plaques may form. The deposits may narrow or block your arteries. These plaques can also rupture, causing a blood clot.

Prevention of Diabetes

The primary strategy to avoiding complications is to prevent blood glucose control to be raising up and it has been shown in major clinical trials show how poor management of diabetes increase the risk of diabetes complication and in the other hand also a good management help to reduce the risk of microvascular and macrovascular complications. In addition, there are other effective ways for people with diabetes to protect themselves regarding complication issues and blood pressure control is also a factor key to preventing both complications in the nearest future. Lowering your blood glucose and cholesterol or by taking your daily dosage and stopping smoking if you do smoke, because it's all effective ways of control the development of macrovascular complications. However it reduce the risk of diabetes complications According to WHO and others researcher who said that there is good report about people suffering of diabetes with a low risk related to diabetes complications and there is other way to help reduce the risk by keeping daily exercises, eating less and loss weight, blood glucose, and cholesterol levels within suggested range and the following are one of the best subjection things you have to do to bring the risk of diabetes complication out of your life.

Blood pressure checks
As a diabetes patient you need to check your blood pressure regular basic and contact or visit your local GP and walk in, because it vital to keep your blood pressure under control of 125/80 to 140/85 if you are diabetes patient, because your blood pressure monitor and your blood glucose control reduce the risk of diabetes complications.

Cholesterol or triglyceride tests
You are advice to have your cholesterol and triglyceride test at least once a year if you are diabetes patients and your aim for total cholesterol less than 4.0 mmol/L and triglycerides

less than 2.0 mmol/L is better to reduce a number that can cause a high cholesterol, including family genetic predisposed and your diet like fatty meats eating, biscuits, cakes to be avoided to help reduce your risk of diabetes complication.

Regular eye checks
People with diabetes disorder should have their eye examination screening by an a qualify optician when you are first diagnosed as diabetes disorder and then every once a years need to be checked up. You can be following up with this screening five years after you been newly diagnosis as diabetes patient just to prevent the onset of complication retinopathy oedema and it is vital to grasp necessary information about diabetes eye check correctly and if your retinopathy or another abnormality is found during your eye tests will be better for early intervention or you will be advised to see your ophthalmologist specialist.

Foot problems and diabetes
The feet of diabetes patients are also at risk of damage when the blood supply in both large and small blood vessels is not supplied blood well to the right direction and the nerve damage called (peripheral neuropathy) can be results to abnormalities and clawed toes would happened. A short blood supply and short nerve function can delay healing of your feet and it increase the risk of infection disease which can cause of non-feeling on the feet, and also cause leg ulcers and foot difficulties to manage.

In a process of your foot care the follow is to look after your feet and if you need to seeing the podiatrist at least once a year to assess your feet health by checking the blood supply, feeling your nerve supply and looking for any changes in your feet structure.

Checking your feet or look for someone to help you if you are unable to check them yourself and look for any cuts that you did recognised during play to be clean and in between the toes of your leg, if any changes you notice, because any early intervention can help prevent complications. For a special treatment or the procedure you need to use moisturiser to sorbolene, rub the dry surface or rough area and cracked skin on your feet. As a matter of fact early treatment can help keeping your feet healthy and also to protecting your feet by wearing comfortable shoes, soft material that fit your foot better.

Skin problems and diabetes
Especially people with diabetes may of them develop a dry skin due to damage to the small blood vessels and nerves system which is a common problem for people diagnose with diabetes. Apart from skin problem, there are also other skin infection regarding diabetes and high blood glucose levels which also causes problem to the skin make the skin to dry and it is vital to keep the skin as healthy as possible and if you left dry skin untreated it can lead to cracks or infections.

To reduce the risk of skin infection
Make sure you control your blood glucose level regular and keep your HbA1c within suggested ranges, so that you will able to reduce the risk of skin infections and advice you will always wear gloves when you are doing a household work or cleaning any solvents. To avoid very hot baths or showers in the house and don't put your feet too close to heaters, and particularly if you are already developed a neuropathy (eye problem) some time you may not be able to feel the passion of your foot and after bathing, use a cream or lotion on your skin immediately to prevent skin inch.

Teeth and gum problems with diabetes
People with diabetes are at higher risk of tooth and gum infections, because the small blood vessels who supplying the gums blood is damage and the dental and gum infections can also lead to high blood glucose levels, because this is a

seriously painful parts. In this case you have to look after your teeth and gums can cause swollen and start to lose your teeth immediately, because with poor oral care can strongly linked to increased risk of heart disease.

Diabetes and Infection

Your immune system helps to prevent your body from infection, because you are a diabetes patients your high blood glucose levels slow down the white blood cells in your body and body can't longer prevent cell that help to fight infection against illness and when white blood cell is affected, your body will now exposed to infection disease. For your white blood cell has been affected and is problem for the immune system to protect your body from infection against your immune system and to reduce high risk of infection is by washing your hands often, keeping your blood glucose levels within the recommended range and get enough sleep each night and get your yearly influenza (flu) immunisation injection to protect yourself.

Thyroid and diabetes problem

People who as been diagnosis with type 1 or type 2 diabetes are at higher risk of thyroid disease and this would result both overactive or underactive thyroid, because thyroid disorders can affect your general health, issues and also affected your blood glucose levels. According to research who said that a diabetic patients have a higher incidence of thyroid disorders when compared with the normal population in worldwide, because patients with autoimmune disorder are also at risk of developing other disease along with diabetes disorder. Meanwhile thyroid disorders are more common in females who are suffering of type 1 diabetic and the rate of thyroiditis in diabetic patients are more likely than that of normal women population. Other number of recent incidence are also reported higher than normal thyroid disorders in type 2 diabetic patients and thyroid can be assessed or detect during HbA1c blood test through your local annual screening by your GP to reduce the onset of thyroid disorder.

Sexual dysfunction and diabetes

Especially the people who are suffering of diabetes have problem of supply blood to the nerve system and blood vessel is damage which cause huge problem or affected function called **sexual dysfunction** (impotence) in men because of inability to achieve erection for sexual performance. This is a common with diabetes people who are on medication or men of all ages and crectile sexual dysfunction is not a disease of its own, but is a sign and symptom of others physical, psychological problem. This happened when physical dysfunction, such as nerve or blood vessel impairment in men or women and there are so many cases that has been reported about sexual dysfunction, but although there no enough evidence base on this issues according to new researcher whether this is directly cause of hormonal changes such as women menopause, or related to diabetes disorder.

Reducing risk of diabetes complications

To reduce the risk of diabetes complication especially when you are at risk related and this can be reduced by keeping blood glucose, blood pressure and cholesterol levels within normal range or by stop smoking, being a healthy weight, reducing alcohol intake, eating healthier foods will help reduce your risk of develop complication. As an diabetes a regularly check-ups is essential to your health and early screening control are important to detect any complications of diabetes.

Diabetes and healthy eating

Healthy eating includes a wide variety of nutritious diet is vital and to avoid snack foods and eating healthy foods with high in fibre would help control your blood pressure, blood glucose and cholesterol levels. To reduce salt intake and follow a recommended food choice guide line can also help promote healthy life.

Alcohol intake and diabetes
You need to put limit into alcohol intake and your lifestyles change could help prevent long standard of complication issues and by not drinking alcohol would be better off per day or if you are a pregnant woman, is advisable not to drink at all or planning to get pregnant either breastfeeding with a new baby born, then you should stop alcohol intake according to WHO discovered.

Diabetes and healthy weight
Diabetes patients need to reduce overweight loss and reduce weight will help lower your blood pressure, blood glucose and cholesterol levels. But people do complain of losing weight, because people want to lose weight do need more encouragement to achieve reduce weight loss and also think about food portion size intake at once.

Diabetes and exercise
Stay physical active is much important if you are diabetes patient and at least 30 minutes of moderate physical activity a day would be better and for weight loss you need a lowest of 60 minutes a day to be perfect shape and if you are unable to participate on normal exercise such as swimming, walking exercise, or gym then consider to see your doctor if you are not comfortable due to your other medical condition that may avoid you from not doing different types of physical activity. Physical activity is one of the best prevention of diabetes complication by keeping time of 30 minute a day walk and doing exercise is vital point to keep your weight in order to help with heart rate and psychological wellbeing.

Smoking and diabetes
Smoking is one of the highest lifestyle risk factor that people with diabetes can develop complications from and smoking can affects all area of circulation by increasing heart rate and high blood pressure, and also damage the small blood vessels thinner during blood flow. Smoking also allows hazardous fatty material to build up in your liver in the body and it can lead to heart attack, stroke and other blood vessel disease and if you are diabetes you smoke you are at high risk of blood pressure and blood glucose levels.

Sleeping patterns
A good sleep both short 6hr and 10hr sleeping a day also contributed to higher risk of developing type 2 diabetes and a short sleep may impair the balance of hormones regulating to food intake and also energy balance. People with diabetes who having long sleep durations may be a sign of sleeping disorder and this can cause obesity and obstructive sleep apnoea syndrome (osa) in future life.

The Diabetes Treatment

According to new research who said that there is no "cure" for any type of diabetes, although with decent management and under control of your diabetes or you're following the recommended treatment would help to prevent the onset of diabetes complication. With good control of your blood sugar levels in the cell that would also help prevent you to have a better long life with diabetes and with the new studies also have shown that good control of blood sugar level is the key to avoid diabetic long-term and short term complications. with type 1 diabetes which requires insulin injection as first treatment of your diabetes management so that it will replaces the missing insulin in the your blood cell and also learn how to balance your insulin within the normal range when eating your food carbohydrate that supplied energy to the body. As diabetes person you need more information that will help you to work with diabetes educator base on care plan to meet your needs in your care team who will assist you managing your diabetes disorder. With type 2 diabetes treatment also base on your blood sugar levels and many diabetes sufferers has been told to changes their lifestyle or to lose more of their weight to prevent diabetes complication and it is also an essential to agree with a diabetes educator team and dietician to help control your blood sugar levels. In some cases first treatment after medication will begins with lifestyles change so as physical exercise, eating balance diet to manage your weight loss. Diabetes treatment may change over time, and it might require oral medication, if you are already on medication or see your doctor every six months to do HbA1c blood test until your blood sugar is in good control or normal range and once it's under control, your medication regime will be reviewed every six months by your GP. Monitoring your blood sugar depend on your treatment plan, you may need to check and record your blood sugar level daily or if you're on insulin, multiple times a day would be better or you should ask your doctor how often you would be check up your blood sugar. Other way round by carefully monitor your blood sugar level is the only way to make sure that your blood sugar level remains within your target range and sometimes, blood sugar levels can be unpredictable or play around. With the help from your diabetes treatment team or professional person you'll learn how your blood sugar level changes in response to food, exercise, alcohol, illness and medication time. In the beginning your diabetes medications and insulin therapy it will help within a month until your blood sugar is under control and your medication regime will be or change if you are type 2 diabetes if your glucose still in higher level. This decision can be made by your GP or professional teams if you had other health condition that you may have to take other medication for, but your doctor might also combine difference drugs classes to help you control your blood sugar levels to normal target range.

People with type 2 diabetes will also achieve a good life successfully and with their target blood sugar levels through a meal diet plan and daily physical exercise will help to normal life expectance with blood glucose control level and make sure you're taking the right dose of insulin to prevent further complication. To avoid complication issues with type 1 diabetes you'll be referred to local hospital specialist, clinic for further investigation, because all doctors, nurses, professional qualify people will give you some advice about how support and how to use self-management procedure with your diabetes at home.

Insulin Taking
Insulin is an essential medication use to managing type 1 diabetes and it helps to control or keep you blood glucose level to normal position. This happened after you have been diagnosis and put you on insulin as soon as possible and the medication is for life term use while to be taken sometimes twice or more times to be taken a day. Taken medication may take a while for your body to amend to it, because you

are taking insulin for the first time and there are different types of insulin and the types of insulin are label in a different category and depend how quicker they active on your system. Some are likely rapid-acting in short-acting and long-acting way, these medication insulin may depend on the category of your depend on your age, eyesight, ability to use injections or pumps in right way would be assess by the professional and how well your blood glucose is controlled to get the target range. Taken insulin injections or insulin pumps, your doctor or diabetes specialist nurse will discussed with you what type of insulin and the safer method to do it.

Side effects of insulin
Your blood sugar levels is already high before you beginning with insulin which would cause you to feel anxious, hungry and shaky when you first taking this insulin, but it only last for short time and go always for shorter period. Checking your blood sugar regular is the best way to improve your sugar levels not to drop too low and the side effect include,

Blurry vision. This is temporary, because as your blood sugar levels go down and this may improve your vision side to see better.

Insulin Therapy and Low Blood Sugar
Being on insulin therapy this can cause you low blood sugar level and you also need to regular monitoring your blood sugar level al time to discovery how the insulin is affecting your blood sugar level.

Insulin injections
You have already had insulin injections in your body through your intravenous vein which is the most common form of the treatment of diabetes type 1 schedule and advised is for you is to inject insulin before morning meals

and this will base on your decision either the small needle or depend of your body intravenous position.

Insulin injection side effects
You will experience redness, swelling and itching at the injection site and changes in your skin, or a build-up in your cell and weight gain.

Portable insulin pumps
This is equipment made up of portable devices which attached to your body or belly with help of waist band and belt round with long design catheter that is programming the constant amount of insulin into your blood stream and these insulin pumps may also be recommended for children under 12 year and also used by people with type 1 diabetes and type 2 diabetes patients.

Insulin pumps side effects
  Headache

  Weight gain

  Hypoglycaemia, or low blood sugar

  Flu

Metformin
Metformin is the first medication prescribed for type 2 diabetes from your GP and it works by refining the sensitivity of your body skins to enable insulin to work effectively in your bloodstream and metformin also used to lowers glucose level in the liver and it may not lower your blood sugar on its own, your doctor may recommend lifestyle changes to losing more weight if gain more weight and becoming more physical active to help reducing you high glucose level. Side effect of metformin - Nausea and diarrhoea are possible side effects of metformin and side effects usually go away as your body gets used to the medicine and if you notice metformin side effect contact

your GP immediately and change of lifestyles could be better to enable you to control your blood sugar level.

Metformin side effects

Fast breath, Fever, Abdominal or stomach pain, diarrhoea.

Sulfonylureas

This type of medication or drugs is special for people with type 2 diabetes treatment plan, because with type 2 diabetes the body doesn't use insulin properly and with diet and exercise it will help control blood sugar levels. Taking sulfonylureas medication and healthy lifestyle, can help improved reduce your risk of developing life-threatening diabetes complications.

Side Effects of Sulfonylureas, dizziness, confusion low blood sugar, skin reactions, sweating, hunger
Weight gain, Dark-coloured urine

Thiazolidinediones

This is just like metformin, these medications help to produce body's skins more sensitive to insulin and with these classes of medications which is also linked to weight gain and seriously side effects, such as an increased risk of heart failure and frequent leg dislocated. Due to a seriously side effect of these medication which might not be the first-choice treatment prescription from your GP when a person has been diagnosis with type 1 diabetes and like the DPP-4 inhibitors are medications also used to reduce blood sugar levels, but they don't produce more side effects to the body or gain weight. These medications help slow your digestion and lower your blood sugar levels and the class of medications isn't frequently recommended for use by your doctor.

Side effect

Receptor agonist's possible side effects include nausea and an increased risk of pancreatitis and eyesight problem, weight gain, skin infection and chest pain.

SGLT2 inhibitors

These are the newest diabetes drugs on the market and it work by preventing the kidneys from reabsorbing sugar into the blood stream or in the body and while using this medication your blood sugar start to excreted through the urine bladder, on examples of this medication include canagliflozin (Invoking) and dapagliflozin.

Side effects
Urinary tract infection
Low blood sugar level
Frequent urination
Yeast infection

Insulin therapy.
With type 1 and type 2 diabetes some people need insulin as well, but insulin therapy is used at last for the treatment of all type if other medication is not working through and today it's often prescribed sooner because of its benefits to patients.

Side Effects
Rash at the site of injection
Low blood sugar and weight gain.
Lumps when too many insulin injections

What is Ketoacidosis

Diabetic ketoacidosis (DKA) is a serious disease that lead to diabetic coma or pass out for a long time and ketoacidosis can occur if the body spends a significant amount of time with too little insulin to refuel the cells of the body and this occurs when the body is unable or short of blood glucose. Because there is not enough insulin in the bloodstream to be use as energy and instead it will break down fat in the cell as an alternative way to get energy usually starving time and these process it becomes a harmful product to the body called ketones in your urine. Ketoacidosis happened sometime especially during a sick period you don't have appetite to eat well and it will result in high ketone in your blood that build up a chemical called ketone acidosis in your body, because you're lack of insulin in your blood cell that causes the body to start breaks down fat somewhere for energy use. In these process a high levels of ketones in the body, which lead to diabetic coma happen and the condition can be very dangerous to life threating. Ketoacidosis affected people with type 1 diabetes than in type 2 diabetes, but is very common to people that have had a surgical removal of the pancreas and if you are experience or develop ketoacidosis you better seek advice from medical doctor for blood test, because it might lead to serious life threating. The high levels of ketones in the bloodstream can poison the body immediately, but can be prevented or been control over it by be aware of the warning signs and symptoms and also checking your urine if feel a very strong smell. It's very important to seek urgent medical attention if someone is displaying the symptoms of the following, **Nausea, vomiting, or abdominal pain** (Vomiting can be caused by many illnesses and if vomiting continuously for more than two hours, contact your health care provider for further investigation.)

Treatment for Diabetic Ketoacidosis

This based on how severity your symptoms are and you may need emergency admission in the ward or intensive care unit and diabetes ketoacidosis is treated in different categories, you may need fluid into your intravenous vein to rehydrate your body, because insulin needed and potassium (minerals needed to recover your dehydration that is lost from the body). You will be also monitored by using blood and urine test to know how well you are responded to treatment or not before discharge you home. In many cases this incidence will take place within 24 hours and although some people may need to remained in the hospital for longer time when you have a combination of several method to abnormal blood sugar and insulin levels or if you're diagnoses with DKA for the first time the doctor might have treatment plan process to keep your ketoacidosis away for a while to avoid repeated and if this incident cause by ordinary infection your investigation test would tell and the necessary treatment would be put in place.

Replacement of Fluid

At the hospital your doctor, physician and qualify nurses will give you fluids to replace the lost of DKA and this fluid need through an IV, because it help for you regain your dehydrated that can cause high blood glucose or low level. The fluids will replace those you've lost through excessive urination, as well as help dilute the excess sugar in your bloodstream.

Insulin therapy

Normally your insulin need to be administer through your intravenous vein until your blood glucose level is balance or fall below 5 to 7mmol (220mg/dL) and when doctor seen your blood level is average range and the doctor will discharge and advised you to avoid the risk of DKA in the nearest future.

Lower than normal range

As diabetes patient if your glucose level lower than normal rage this can cause the level of electrolytes in body cell to break down and electrolytes in your body are called electrically charged or current help your body, heart and nerves to function properly and lose of replacement of electrolytes is done through IV in your body whenever you're being hospitalised.

Electrolyte replacement

Electrolytes are minerals in your blood that carry an electric charger, such as sodium, potassium and chloride and if this absence, insulin can lower the level of several electrolytes in the body. You'll also receive electrolytes through a vein to help keep your heart, muscles and nerve cells functioning normal.

Insulin therapy

Insulin reverses the processes that cause diabetic ketoacidosis. In addition to fluids and electrolytes, you'll receive insulin therapy as a treatment through the vein. When your blood sugar level falls below 240 mg/dL (13.3 mmol/L) and your blood is no longer acidic, you may be able to stop intravenous insulin therapy and resume your normal insulin treatment.

Glaucoma

Glaucoma damage to the optical nerve in the eye ball and this optic nerve is the one that is connected from the eyes to the brain and in adult with diabetes have a huge incident double risk of glaucoma than the normal population without diabetes. Diabetic retinopathy is known as number one killer or the cause to diabetes blindness and because you already have a visual disability, which affected in small blood vessel that damage to the back layer of the eye, that would lead to progressive loss of vision and even leading to blindness immediately.

Symptoms

The eye blurred vision is one of the symptoms and in the other hand, another symptoms can also be appearing during these period and there are some symptoms that may occur this might need urgent intervention, because without concern it can result blindness. If you are unfortunate to have flashes of light, blots and dots or felt part of your vision is missing, seek urgent medical advice.

Treatment

A good control of your body metabolic can also delay the onset of blindness if you are diabetes patients and early treatment of vision detect can prevent retinopathy condition to be worst. What happened when blood vessel is leaking in the eyes of diabetes patients you may need laser photocoagulation to prevent the loss of your eye vision.

What is Hyperglycaemia

Hyperglycaemia occurs when people with diabetes have too much sugar in their blood cell and is also a term use to expressing high blood glucose level in the blood cell and is also defined by WHO when blood glucose levels is greater than 10.0 mmol/L (156 mg/dl). With poor management of glucose level which can cause damage to your internal organs, but symptoms may not develop until blood glucose levels exceed 10 to 20 mmol/L sometime this might take several time in your body before it happened. Hyperglycaemia (hyper) means having high blood glucose levels than the target rate if you consider yourself as a diabetes patients and with consistently high blood glucose levels can be dangerous when left untreated. The underlying cause of hyperglycaemia will usually classify as lack of insulin that producing cells in the pancreas when the body is stimulated resistance to insulin treatment or by missing a dose of diabetic medication for few days can cause hyperglycaemia. In some cases develop a eating habit or more carbohydrates intake as usual, your body would reacted to it or any other illness or being mentally unwell and emotionally distress can cause to hyperglycaemia if you are diabetes person.

To preventing hyperglycaemia

To preventing hyperglycaemia for people with a diabetes type and taking a good control or self-monitoring of blood glucose levels daily it will help to prevent the onset of consciousness, coma or stroke. For those who has not been diagnosed with any diabetes or any symptoms of hyperglycaemia need to be reported to local doctor immediately so that they will do on investigation test for diabetes or other condition. Having other conditions which can also cause hyperglycaemia crisis should be also reported to your local clinic for the first time to prevent the onset of emergency of your high glucose level.

While a frequently hyperglycaemia by patients can be review treatment plan.

Manage your carbs, As an diabetes person u don't' consume too much carbohydrate at ago during meal time and try stay with recommendation plan from doctor or dietician and be smart to draw up your plan of action if your blood glucose level get to a certain stage. Being reliable about your time and amount of meals you consumed at a goals that is order way to prevent hyperglycaemia as patients or if you identify a sign warning.

Wearing a medical identification (ID), because many people with diabetes, particularly those who use a regular insulin, should have a medical ID on them at all times in case of crisis situation or if any other incidents happen with severe hypoglycaemic or hyperglycaemia episode. This medical ID that can give someone information about the person's health situation regarding been diabetes person. Advised, emergency medical trained specialist or professional need to check for medical ID to make it easier for someone who can't speak for themselves during crisis period of time.

Untreated hyperglycaemia ketoacidosis.

Hyperglycaemia can be a seriously issues if you don't treat it early and it's essential to treat as soon as early if detect if you fail to recognise hyperglycaemia a ketoacidosis (diabetic coma) can be happened immediately. Ketoacidosis is progresses when your body doesn't produce sufficiency insulin to the cell and without insulin, your body can't use glucose (sugar) for fuel and them your body start breaks down fats to use as energy in the body. What happen during ketoacidosis, is that when your body breaks down fats, waste products called ketones are produced to use as energy and because your body cannot bear large amounts of ketones in the body and kidney will try to get rid of them through the urine track system. Unfortunately, the body cannot release all the ketones through your waste product, they it will build up in your bloodstream, which can lead to ketoacidosis.

Hypoglycaemia Of Diabetes

Hypoglycaemia is defined as blood glucose level fall below 4mmol/L and hypos can happen when diabetes patients is untreated without no medication or someone has other condition and it also happen when someone on others diabetes medication called sulfonylureas medication. Hypos should be treated immediately and left untreated could be worse or leading to patients having experience of unconscious or in comma, stroke, because there is no enough insulin to the cell, delayed, missed meal carbohydrate, unplanned exercise, drinking alcohol without food can cause hypoglycaemia symptoms. According to the new researcher who said that there is no evident base whatever causes or warning signs of hypoglycaemia when are taking right insulin or other oral medications for your diabetes and this reaction occur when you are short of glucose in the cell. A hypoglycaemic reaction usually happened suddenly without any sign and symptoms warning, especially when your meal is delayed and patients need also to recognise their own side infect of any insulin reaction at all time. Some example if someone begins to feel any symptoms or think your blood glucose may be too low, check your blood level immediately using a blood glucose test BM machine and if less than 70 mg/dl 3.0mmol, then you are probably having a hypoglycaemic reaction. The good news is be aware of the early sign of hypoglycaemia reaction known as low blood glucose and the used of glucose gel or sweet honey, fruit juice as first treatment when someone experience hypoglycaemia reaction. If happened dial 999 and don't give food or drink to someone who is unconscious or a persists seizure for more than 5 minutes and several hypos can be handle with glucagon gel or look if glucagon injection kits is available.

The causes of hypoglycaemia

A diabetes medication is the main factors that can cause hypoglycaemia to diabetes patients and many number of other factors can contributed to increase the risk of hypos to patients. There are other most common causes of hypoglycaemia when insulin is too much in the body or long stayed exercise, or not eating enough food.

What are the symptoms of hypoglycaemia

There are two major types of hypoglycaemia symptoms, the Neurogenic are the result of the beginning sympatric nervous system when you see blood glucose drop to lower level and the reaction become sweating, shakiness, anxiety, a sensation of hunger, tingling and tachycardia (heart) attack can take place. The Neuroglycopenic symptoms will arise when there is no insufficient blood glucose in the blood cell to use as fuel energy to the brain, include, weakness, tiredness, dizziness; inappropriate behaviour. During the prolonged or severe hypoglycaemia occur to you it will dysfunction the brain which lead to coma or death and people with low glucose levels sometime they have little awareness of the symptoms and with others people normal glucose levels may also display their hypoglycaemic symptoms.

Diagnosis of hypoglycaemia

By express diagnosis with immediate treatment is vital to any patient who has been suspected hypoglycaemia, regardless of your illness and the patients would be recognised for his symptomatic display and should be documented as a low blood sugar level or other condition. The elderly persons known as a patients of concerns who exhibit fewer symptoms of hypoglycaemia when still dependant of any medication or because of their onset of plasma glucose level is lower at all presentation. For further advised if anybody who has a hypoglycaemic attack, because it does not know why, should contacted doctor as soon as possible and patients record medical history should be check immediately to known whether there have been any recent involved in heavy drinking.

Treatment of hypoglycaemia

Prevention of hypoglycaemia is a major key to reducing the risk for diabetic coma, stroke and to manage your diabetes accordingly to your GP instruction and especially why type 1 diabetes also puts more people at a higher risk for coma crisis and people suffering of type 2 are also at risk of developing hypoglycaemia, but incident are not common.

Glucose injection. Inject glucose into intravenous infusion in a large vein as requested and a good close monitor is needed in case of any other meds administer and if a patient develop hypoglycemia which cause by use of antidiabetic drug and this can be monitor or transferred immediately to the hospital when continue persist for longer time or hours.

Self-monitor blood glucose. As a diabetes patient this is something you should always do to prevent hypoglycemia to occur, but in previous cases you have hypoglycemia episodes before the doctor may check your blood glucose level throughout the day until your glucose level is well monitor.

To be carrying your glucose tablets. A diabetes person should be carry your glucose tablet along with your sweetness, cheese and candy with you away and you may also want to keep your snack foods on hand bag to help prevent or delay hypoglycemia situation.

Working with dietician. The most important is to adjust your meal plan to wash out what you eat every day is vital in your blood sugar level and special dietician can explained what you can eat to help balance or stabilise your healthy lifestyle for your glucose level to be on a safer side.

Exercise: A regular exercise is an effective way to control your blood sugar, but advice too much physical activity can consume excess glucose in your body and what happen if a person with severe hyperglycemia and ketones is finds in the urine test, the person should avoid daily exercise, because it will breaks down more fats in your body to use as energy and it might speed up ketoacidosis to poison your blood cells and end up in coma, because your blood mix with toxic acid already in the blood.

Eating diet: Eating less during mealtimes and snacking less during the day or night and keep well focusing on a low fat sugar foods to help reduce the amount of blood glucose at time, special diabetic food pack or a dietician can help a person adapt their diet in healthful ways.

Medications: A doctor might referred you to change the time or to look at different types of medication or the insulin a person is taking if they are not reducing blood sugar level the healthcare professional or doctor need to find a way to increase dosage.

Adjustment to your insulin dose. To control your hyperglycemia person have to adjust to your insulin program, because a short acting insulin can help control hyperglycemia and you can use supplement as an extra dose of insulin to help you control your high blood sugar level and asked your healthcare professional or the doctor how often you need an insulin supplement if continue having high blood sugar.

Feeling Sick. If you are feeling sick or unwell vomiting you must contact your doctor or healthcare team for more advice to understand how different treatments can help keep your glucose levels within your goal range.

Other Treatments for hypoglycaemia.

A mild case of hypoglycaemia can be treated through eating or drinking 15-20g of fast acting carbohydrate such as glucose tablets, sweets, sugary fizzy drinks or fruit juice and a table spoon of honey. Severe hypoglycaemia may require an ambulance for example if loss of consciousness occurs or a seizure persists for more than 5 minutes and it can be treated with glucagon if a glucagon injection kit is available in your environment or car.

Summary

Pancreas is the major fundamental issues of diabetes mulitus with type 1 that autoimmune system is not producing insulin to the cell why because the beta cell has been damaged and the body is unable to produce any insulin to the cell and while type 2 diabetes which supply a little insulin to cell, but not enough to use as energy.

The treatment and self-management plan is to keep your diabetes and glucose level in a good shape to prevent complication and also food that contain sugary should be avoided, but you can still enjoy your favourite food and plan to limit too much sugar intake. In fact you must also cut down on setting carbs and select the type of carbohydrates food you consume at a time. To prevent you might need a diabetic special meals plan as recommended from WHO and following up the principle of healthy eating to minimise a portion size of food consume daily to enable you get the best key to reduce your high glucose level. The complication of diabetes known as Micro and Macrovascular base on high and low blood build up in the blood cell and micro is the cause of diabetic retinopathy disease (eye) is the leading eye blindness and macrovascular disease CVD referred to heart and stroke and this is also cause by hyperglycaemia that is affected people with diabetes than the general population.

As diabetes patients food that is high in protein is the best, but eating too much protein or animal protein may cause insulin resistance and healthy diet to diabetes patients, like protein, carbohydrates, and fats food are the best food to control your blood sugar level. In other cases we still need this three type of protein in our life to be function with.

As an diabetes patients work hard to knowing your diabetes **ABCs** management will help you manage your blood sugar level, blood pressure, and cholesterol and eventually stop smoking will also help you manage your diabetes mellitus and to work toward your **ABCs** goals it will help lower your diabetes complication.

Diabetes ABCs Goals,

A- for the A1c blood test, The A1C blood test is shows your average blood sugar level over the past 2-3 months and A1c also know as HbA1c Haemoglobin use for blood test to diagnose type 1 and type 2 and is also use to monitor how well you're managing you diabetes treatment.

B- for Blood pressure monitor, The goal for diabetes patient is to monitor their blood pressure and an expected average reading bellow is 140/90 mm Hg when you are diabetes.

C- for Cholesterol test, A diabetes patient should have cholesterol and triglycerides check, because there are bad cholesterol in the blood cell and they can build up in your blood vessels and cause blockage of glucose circulation and some people are more likely to get heart disease in the future. Example if you are above 35/50 years of age, you may have the risk because of your age and medication for heart health wise.

S- for Stop smoking, As an diabetes person is better not to smoke at all, because smoking narrow your blood vessels the vessel makes your heart work more double than normal population and is a good idea to quit smoking, because it improve and lower the risk of heart attack, stroke, nerve disease or amputation.

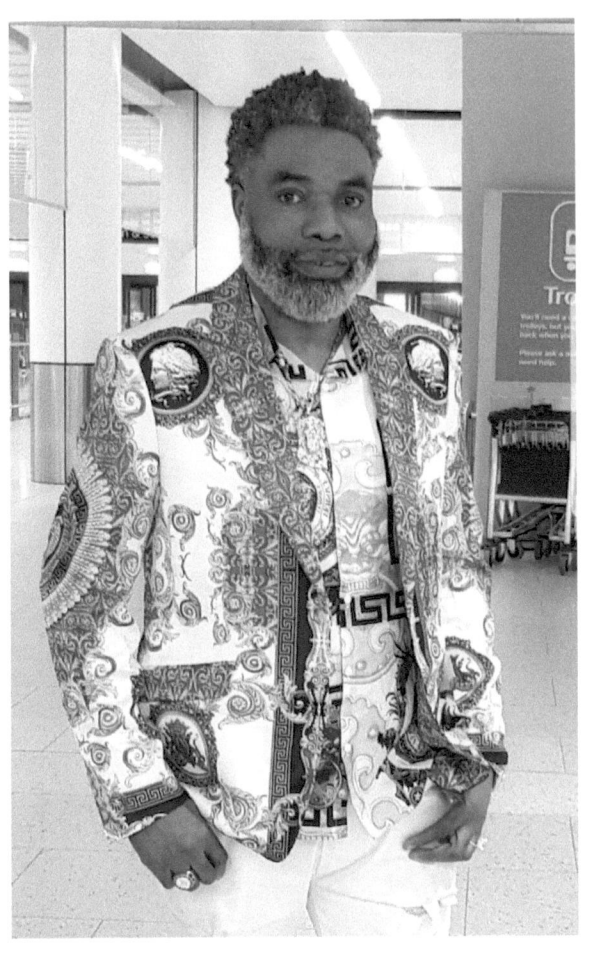

GODWIN MILLINGTON

www.ingramcontent.com/pod-product-compliance
Ingram Content Group UK Ltd.
Pitfield, Milton Keynes, MK11 3LW, UK
UKHW042001230426
12048UKWH00009B/460